Precancerous Lesions
of the Gastrointestinal Tract

Precancerous Lesions of the Gastrointestinal Tract

A Histological Classification

BASIL C. MORSON, VRD, DM, FRCS, FRCP, FRCPath

Head, World Health Organization Collaborating Centre
for Histological Classification of Alimentary Tract Tumours
and Precancerous Lesions, Pathology Department,
St Mark's Hospital, London, England

AND

JEREMY R. JASS, BSc, MD, MRCPath

Senior Lecturer and Honorary Consultant in Histopathology,
Westminster Medical School, London, England

IN COLLABORATION WITH

LESLIE H. SOBIN, MD, FRCPath

Head, World Health Organization Collaborating Center for
International Histological Classification of Tumors,
Armed Forces Institute of Pathology, Washington, DC, USA

1985

Baillière Tindall London Philadelphia Toronto
Mexico City Rio de Janeiro Sydney Tokyo Hong Kong

Baillière Tindall   1 St Anne's Road
W. B. Saunders   Eastbourne, East Sussex BN21 3UN, England

West Washington Square
Philadelphia, PA 19105, USA

1 Goldthorne Avenue
Toronto, Ontario M8Z 5T9, Canada

Apartado 26370—Cedro 512
Mexico 4, DF Mexico

Rua Evaristo da Veiga 55, 20° andar
Rio de Janeiro—RJ, Brazil

ABP Australia Ltd, 44 Waterloo Road
North Ryde, NSW 2113, Australia

Ichibancho Central Building, 22–1 Ichibancho
Chiyoda-ku, Tokyo 102, Japan

10/fl, Inter-Continental Plaza, 94 Granville Road
Tsim Sha Tsui East, Kowloon, Hong Kong

First published 1985

Photoset by Paston Press, Norwich
Printed and bound in Italy
by G. Canale & C. S.p.A, Turin

British Library Cataloguing in Publication Data

Morson, Basil C.
   Precancerous lesions of the gastrointestinal
   tract.
   1. Digestive organs—Cancer
   2. Precancerous conditions
   I. Title   II. Jass, Jeremy R.   III. Sobin, L. H.
   616.99′2307   RC280.D5

ISBN 0-7020-1053-7 (book)
ISBN 0-7020-1054-5 (transparencies)

Contents

Contents

Anal Canal 14
A. Dysplasia and carcinoma-in-situ, 14
B. Dysplasia in leukoplakia, 14

Anal Margin 14
A. Dysplasia, 14
B. Condyloma acuminatum (viral wart), 14
C. Paget's disease, 15
D. Bowen's disease, 15

Preface

In 1976 the World Health Organization established a Collaborating Centre in the Pathology Department of St Mark's Hospital, London for the study of precancerous lesions and conditions of the alimentary tract (oesophagus to anus). The Centre has a large collection of precancerous lesions of the oesophagus, stomach, duodenum and small intestine, appendix, colorectum and anal region which have been obtained from the files of the Pathology Department of St Mark's Hospital as well as from many outside sources. We are grateful to those pathologists from all parts of the world, too numerous to mention by name, who have donated material. We also wish to express our special gratitude to Dr H. J. R. Bussey for his administrative and professional support.

At a first meeting of the Centre held at the Ciba Foundation in London in July 1978, precancerous lesions of the stomach were discussed and the results were subsequently published in 1980 (*Journal of Clinical Pathology* 33: 711–721). The work of the Centre on colorectal adenomas was published in 1982 (*Journal of Clinical Pathology* 35: 830–841).

The present publication aims at bringing together the wide variety of lesions associated with an increased risk of developing into cancer, to name and classify them in an orderly, internationally acceptable manner, and to define and illustrate them histologically. This publication is not intended to serve as a textbook but rather to promote the adoption of a uniform terminology and categorization of precancerous lesions that will facilitate and improve communication among cancer workers. For this reason the literature references have intentionally been kept to a minimum and readers are referred to standard works on the subject for extensive bibliographies. It will of course be appreciated that the classification reflects the present state of knowledge and modifications are almost certain to be needed as experience accumulates. Although the present classification necessarily represents a view from which some pathologists may wish to dissent, it is nevertheless hoped that in the interests of international cooperation all pathologists will try to use the classification as put forward. Criticisms and suggestions for improvement will be welcome. These should be sent to the Director, World Health Organization Collaborating Centre for the Histological Classification of Precancerous Lesions of the Alimentary Tract, St Mark's Hospital, London EC1V 2PS, England.

The colour photomicrographs appearing in this book are also available as a collection of transparencies intended for teaching purposes. These may be obtained by writing to the Publishers, Baillière Tindall, or its affiliated companies worldwide (see page iv).

Finally, we should like to express our gratitude to the Publishers, as represented by Geoffrey Smaldon, Cliff Morgan, David Manson and David Inglis, for their care and efficiency throughout the concluding stages of preparation of the manuscript and the speedy production of this book.

BASIL C. MORSON
JEREMY R. JASS

Introduction

A precancerous *lesion* is a histopathological abnormality in which cancer is more likely to occur than in its apparently normal counterpart (Morson et al, 1980). It is distinguished from a precancerous *condition*, which is a clinical state associated with a significantly increased risk of cancer.

The term 'precancerous' does not imply the inevitability of developing a malignant lesion. It is rather a marker of an increased probability or risk of malignant change. Nor is it implied that all cancers must necessarily develop within a precancerous lesion.

Lesions thought to be associated with an increased cancer risk for the individual patient frequently exhibit an epithelial alteration known as dysplasia (synonymous with intraepithelial neoplasia). This histological abnormality is characterized by cytological atypia, aberrant differentiation and disorganized architecture. Dysplasia occurs in both squamous and columnar epithelium and is recognized in routine histological preparations. Special techniques involving histochemistry, electron microscopy and cytogenetics can be used for its detailed study, but its diagnosis and assessment are based mainly on conventional haematoxylin and eosin stained paraffin sections.

The risk of cancer developing depends on the grade or severity of the dysplasia. High grade or severe dysplasia is closest to cancer, lacking only the property of invasion. Lesser forms may be divided into mild and moderate; alternatively, the term 'low grade' may be preferred. Interpretation is also influenced by the organ under consideration and the clinical and pathological context pertaining to the lesion, such as the presence of irritation, ulceration, inflammation or regeneration.

The recognition of dysplasia is not necessarily straightforward. Particular problems are the distinction between regenerative, inflammatory and reactive change and genuine dysplasia, and the separation of severe dysplasia and invasive carcinoma. In addition, there are several disorders of differentiation whose nature is poorly understood, e.g. incomplete intestinal metaplasia in the stomach and incomplete maturation in inflammatory bowel disease.

The histological recognition of dysplasia is of clinical importance, but little is known of the magnitude of risk associated with this lesion, particularly in an individual case. Follow-up is important, both to establish the biological behaviour of the lesion and for the sake of the patient. Over-diagnosis should be avoided as it will burden both clinician and patient and result in disenchantment with the term. Under-diagnosis will undermine the point of the exercise—the prevention and early detection of carcinoma.

Some of the lesions that will be presented are poorly documented and others have only recently been described. For this reason the text will include not only descriptions of the histology, but also a few key references and some indication of the clinical background and relevance of the lesion.

Histological Classification of Precancerous Lesions of the Gastrointestinal Tract

OESOPHAGUS

A. Chronic oesophagitis (Figs. 1–5)

This lesion may be important in the pathogenesis of squamous cell carcinoma, but is not specific enough to serve as a useful premalignant marker. An unusual distribution, with involvement of the mid-oesophagus, is seen in high risk communities in Iran and China (Muñoz et al, 1982). Clear cell acanthosis or hyperplasia is also seen in these high risk groups, but again is too common to be of practical importance (Fig. 2). Atrophy may be an intermediate step between chronic oesophagitis and frank dysplasia (Fig. 3). Chronic oesophagitis is characterized by papillomatosis, infiltration by lymphocytes and plasma cells, and proliferation and dilatation of blood vessels of the epithelium and submucosa (Fig. 2). Clear cell acanthosis is a thickening of the epithelium by swollen clear cells that are usually PAS negative.

B. Dysplasia and carcinoma-in-situ (Figs. 6–15)

Dysplasia within the squamous epithelium of the oesophagus is similar to the more extensively investigated lesion encountered in the uterine cervix (Barge et al, 1981). The hallmark of this lesion is an abnormal or dyskaryotic nucleus, which is enlarged and hyperchromatic. In mild dysplasia, such nuclei are limited to the basal zone and, superficially, cytoplasmic differentiation is evident (Fig. 6). With increasing grades of dysplasia, there is a progressive increase in the proportion of atypical basal cells until the entire thickness of the mucosa is replaced (carcinoma-in-situ) (Figs. 7 and 8). Mitoses are numerous. This neoplastic proliferation is accompanied by vertical compression of the underlying stroma, so that vascularized finger-like processes extend close to the surface (Fig. 8). Glycogenation decreases with increasing grades of dysplasia, and carcinoma-in-situ is associated with an absence of glycogen (Figs. 13–15). This finding is utilized in the iodine test for the macroscopic demonstration of carcinoma-in-situ (Mandard et al, 1980). Dysplasia and carcinoma-in-situ are frequently multifocal lesions (Ushigome et al, 1967).

Dysplasia may be difficult to distinguish from the reactive and regenerative changes associated with reflux oesophagitis, in which there is also hyperplasia of the basal cell layer accompanied by nuclear pleomorphism, hyperchromatism, an increased mitotic index, and both thinning and elongation of the papillae (Figs. 10,

3

27 and 28). In true dysplasia, the nuclear characteristics are essentially those of malignancy.

Dysplasia and carcinoma-in-situ in squamous mucosa are more likely to occur in patients with precancerous conditions. These include achalasia, tylosis, the Paterson–Brown–Kelly (Plummer–Vinson) syndrome, coeliac disease (O'Brien et al, 1983) and lye strictures.

There is no evidence that precancerous leukoplakia, as seen in the mouth or vulva, occurs in the oesophagus. White plaques in the oesophagus may be associated with a variety of lesions, including oesophagitis, moniliasis, glycogenic acanthosis, lichen planus (Figs. 4 and 5) and the clear cell acanthosis of chronic oesophagitis (Fig. 2). When accompanied by superficial hyperkeratosis, dysplasia and carcinoma-in-situ may present as a white plaque (Figs. 7 and 8).

Carcinoma has occasionally been noted to supervene in cases of oral lichen planus (Andreasen, 1968). The risk to patients with oesophageal involvement is unknown, but is unlikely to be high.

C. Barrett's oesophagus (Figs. 16–26)

This is defined as the presence of columnar epithelium within the lower oesophagus. Most workers regard this lesion as an acquired heterotopia or metaplasia consequent upon reflux oesophagitis (Trier and Curtis, 1983). Three types of columnar epithelium have been observed, either singly or in combination (Paull et al, 1976):

1. Junctional or cardiac type (Fig. 16)
2. Fundic type with parietal and chief cells (Fig. 17)
3. Specialized or intestinal (Figs. 18–21)

The specialized mucosa has a villiform surface which is lined by goblet cells and mucus-secreting columnar cells and includes glands lined by cuboidal seromucinous cells. Paneth cells, endocrine cells and absorptive-type cells can be found but are not conspicuous. The columnar mucous cells (or principal cells) show evidence of aberrant differentiation both histochemically and at the ultrastructural level (Trier, 1970; Berenson et al, 1974; Ozzello et al, 1977). Specialized epithelium, which is similar to incomplete intestinal metaplasia described in the stomach (Jass, 1981), may account for the increased malignant risk associated with Barrett's oesophagus.

Dysplasia in Barrett's oesophagus resembles gastric dysplasia histologically (see below) (Figs. 22–26). Dysplasia is more likely to arise in the specialized epithelium than in either the cardiac or fundic types (Trier and Curtis, 1983) (Figs. 24 and 25). The presence of dysplasia in Barrett's oesophagus selectively increases the malignant potential of the lesion (Berenson et al, 1978).

D. Lesions simulating dysplasia (Figs. 27–29)

1. *Inflammatory and reactive lesions:* In the presence of acute inflammation, particularly with ulceration, the squamous (or columnar) epithelium may display cellular and architectural changes that can simulate dysplasia (Fig. 27). Loss of cell cohesion in early

ulceration may resemble carcinoma. The multinucleate cells in herpesvirus oesophagitis can be a cause of misinterpretation (McKay and Day, 1983).

2. *Regenerative changes:* The squamous (or columnar) epithelium that is relining an ulcer or erosion can show basophilia, an increased nuclear/cytoplasmic ratio, loss of normal differentiation and disorganization that may simulate dysplasia or carcinoma-in-situ (Figs. 27, 28 and 67).

3. *Radiation changes:* Patients who have received radiotherapy to the chest, e.g. for Hodgkin's disease, may develop inflammatory and ulcerative oesophageal lesions with bizarre fibroblasts and endothelial cells. These may simulate dysplastic or even invasive cells (Berthrong and Fajardo, 1981). Little is known about the natural history and malignant potential of these lesions (Fig. 29).

The assessment of dysplasia in the above circumstances is very difficult and must be carried out with caution.

STOMACH

A. Chronic atrophic gastritis (Figs. 30–33)

The main histological features are a degree of chronic inflammation, fibrosis of the lamina propria, atrophy of gastric glands, pyloric metaplasia, intestinal metaplasia and less commonly dysplasia. Several clinical settings are associated with this lesion, including pernicious anaemia, hypersecretion of acid, bile reflux, gastric surgery and as yet undisclosed environmental influences in, for example, populations at a high risk of developing gastric carcinoma. The distribution of the lesion varies according to the cause. Patients with chronic atrophic gastritis are at an increased risk of developing gastric cancer; indeed most cancers develop on the basis of this lesion. However, intestinal metaplasia and dysplasia are the epithelial changes which statistically most predispose to malignancy (see below).

B. Intestinal metaplasia (Figs. 33–40)

Intestinal metaplasia (IM) may be complete, i.e. mature, when it closely resembles normal small intestine or incomplete when full intestinal differentiation is not achieved. Mature IM is composed of goblet cells secreting mainly sialomucins (see Table 1), brightly

Table 1 Guide to mucin histochemistry (Filipe and Lake, 1983).

Method	Colour	Interpretation
Diastase periodic acid–Schiff	Red	Neutral mucins and some acid mucins
Alcian blue pH 2.5	Blue	Acid mucins (sialomucins and sulphomucins)
Alcian blue pH 1.0	Blue	Sulphomucins
High iron diamine	Brown	Sulphomucins

eosinophilic columnar absorptive cells with a well-developed brush border, and Paneth cells at the crypt base (Figs. 33, 34, 37 and 38). Endocrine cells, appropriate to small intestine, are also present. The crypts are simple tubular structures with little branching or cyst formation. Incomplete IM may be subdivided into two types. Firstly, goblet cells may be scattered amongst apparently normal gastric foveolar cells (simple goblet cell metaplasia) (Fig. 20). Secondly, the goblet cells may be bordered by columnar cells showing ambiguous differentiation and secreting acid and neutral mucins in varying combinations, but often with sulphomucins predominating (Jass, 1980) (Fig. 40). These cells may show a partially developed brush border and are taller and more crowded than the absorptive cells of complete IM. Their nuclei are slightly enlarged and vesicular. The crypts are often lengthened with papillary infolding and branching (Figs. 35 and 36). The underlying glands frequently show cystic change. Paneth cells are few or absent (Fig. 35). This variant of IM is frequently seen bordering gastric carcinomas and within the entity of IM is regarded as a more selective marker of premalignant change (Jass, 1980; Sipponen et al, 1980; Segura and Montero, 1983). However, its precise role in the histogenesis of gastric cancer is not known. Complete IM is too prevalent to serve as a specific precancerous marker in clinical practice, even in low risk areas.

C. Dysplasia (Figs. 41–51)

Dysplasia arises either in flat mucosa affected by chronic gastritis or within raised lesions or polyps (see below) (Morson et al, 1980). Dysplasia cannot be fully evaluated except in the light of the clinical setting responsible for its presence. It arises mainly in metaplastic epithelium, but also in gastric epithelium (Morson et al, 1980). It is frequently possible to demonstrate a continuum between the incomplete form of intestinal metaplasia and dysplasia (Jass, 1983). The lesion is more difficult to diagnose when it arises in flat mucosa since villous or budding tubular structures, which are so characteristic of adenomatous epithelium, may not be apparent (Nagayo, 1981).

Two main types of dysplasia have been described (Cuello et al, 1979; Jass, 1983). In the first, the crypts are lined by columnar cells with darkly staining amphophilic cytoplasm (Fig. 48). The nuclei are elongated, hyperchromatic and pseudostratified (Fig. 49). The cells often secrete small amounts of apical sulphomucin (Figs. 59 and 60). Paneth cells may be absent or misplaced. In the second type, the columnar cells are pale and eosinophilic and may show a partially developed brush border as well as small numbers of apical mucin droplets. Goblet cells may be present but reduced in number and often inverted or malpositioned. Paneth cells are absent. The nuclei are round to ovoid and vesicular with a prominent nucleolus (Figs. 41–47). The intense nuclear crowding and pseudostratification of the first type of dysplasia is not in evidence. Forms intermediate between the two types are commonly seen.

Grading dysplasia into mild, moderate and severe should be carried out in an attempt to quantify the magnitude of risk (Oehlert et al, 1979; Morson et al, 1980). This exercise is subjective and it must be accepted that experience and personal preference will influence the wording of the histological report. However, some uniformity in reporting is needed if the results of different centres are to be compared. Severe dysplasia refers to lesions that closely resemble carcinoma, but do not show invasion. Mild dysplasia is the mildest degree of change that can be confidently diagnosed as dysplasia. It is recognized by a combination of architectural changes, reduction in mucus secretion, and elongation and crowding of nuclei. However, the nuclear/cytoplasmic ratio is little increased, polarity is easily discerned, and there is little variation in nuclear size and shape. Moderate dysplasia lies between these extremes, showing more nuclear abnormalities than mild dysplasia but falling short of severe dysplasia.

The main diagnostic problems are the distinction between reactive and regenerative change and dysplasia (see below), and between severe dysplasia and intramucosal carcinoma. The latter is an important distinction because the diagnosis of intramucosal carcinoma demands surgical intervention, whereas severe dysplasia implies the need for close follow-up only. Intramucosal carcinoma should only be diagnosed if invasion of the lamina propria is demonstrated. In practice, when dysplasia is so severe that a diagnosis of carcinoma-in-situ is entertained, e.g. with intratubular back-to-back gland formation, further investigation will usually reveal frankly invasive carcinoma. Thus a stage of carcinoma-in-situ is rarely seen in the stomach in isolation.

D. Adenoma (Figs. 52–62)

Adenomas are circumscribed lesions composed of dysplastic epithelium (Ming, 1977). The junction with surrounding non-neoplastic epithelium is abrupt (Figs. 54 and 58). The latter is rarely normal, however, showing the changes of chronic gastritis and usually intestinal metaplasia (most often the incomplete type) (Fig. 54). Epithelial dysplasia is the same whether it occurs in raised, flat or even depressed mucosa. Thus it is the grade of the dysplasia and not its elevation that is responsible for the increased risk of malignant change. However, a villous growth pattern may add to this risk, if only by increasing the area of dysplasia.

Most gastric adenomas show a villous or a tubulovillous growth pattern and are sessile rather than pedunculated (Figs. 55–62). Some tubular types show only slight elevation if at all (Figs. 52 and 53). These have been well documented in Japanese literature and referred to as atypical epithelium, flat adenomas or borderline lesions (Sugano et al, 1971; Nagayo, 1971). The latter term has unfortunately been used with different meanings and is best avoided. Adenomatous dysplasia need not occupy the entire thickness of the mucosa. Pyloric-type glands, often cystically dilated, may be present in the lower half of the lesion (Nagayo, 1981).

E. Dysplasia in hyperplastic (regenerative, hyperplasiogenous) polyps (Figs. 63–66)

These are composed of focally polypoid and somewhat disorganized gastric-type epithelium, with or without goblet cell metaplasia (Elster, 1976; Ming, 1977). Dysplasia and malignant change have been described but only very rarely (Kamiya et al, 1981). The possession of multiple hyperplastic polyps may confer a very small increased cancer risk (Tomasulo, 1971), but no adequate explanation for this observation in terms of a histogenetic sequence has been formulated (Figs. 63–66).

F. Gastric ulcer (Figs. 67 and 68)

The relationship between gastric ulcer and gastric carcinoma is complex. The observed coincidence of these lesions is likely to be higher than expected, because both occur in stomachs affected by chronic gastritis. In addition, the actively regenerating epithelium adjacent to an ulcer may be more unstable than normal epithelium (Figs. 67 and 68). Furthermore, peptic ulceration may occur in an intramucosal carcinoma and the result may be difficult to distinguish from an 'ulcer-cancer'.

Ulcer-cancer (i.e. a carcinoma developing in the mucosa around the edge of a chronic peptic ulcer) is infrequent, probably accounting for no more than 1% of gastric carcinomas. The epithelium adjacent to any ulcer should always be examined with care.

G. Dysplasia in Ménétrier's disease (Figs. 69 and 70)

The main pathological features of Ménétrier's disease are rugal hypertrophy due to marked crypt hyperplasia with cystic dilatation of glands and upwards extension of the muscularis mucosae into the lamina propria (Figs. 69 and 70). Gastric carcinoma has been described as a complication of Ménétrier's disease, but its precise histogenesis is not understood and the magnitude of risk is unknown (Morson et al, 1980). Intestinal metaplasia and dysplasia have been documented in this condition.

H. Lesions simulating dysplasia (Figs. 71–74)

When chronic gastritis and the other lesions listed above are complicated by active inflammation, the foveolar epithelium may show regenerative changes which should be distinguished from true dysplasia. Mucin secretion is decreased, though there is little or no qualitative alteration. The cytoplasm is dark and amphophilic with H&E and the nuclei are enlarged and hyperchromatic, but pseudostratification is not marked. The presence of infiltrating neutrophils and the absence of glandular architectural alterations further facilitate the diagnosis of reactive and regenerative change (Figs. 71–73).

Cystic dilatation of deep glands occurs in chronic cystic gastritis (gastritis cystica profunda) (Franzin and Novelli, 1981) (Fig. 32). In the absence of other epithelial alterations, particularly dysplasia, this event probably does not confer a significant cancerous risk, though the deeply situated glands may mimic invasion. Such glands may be lined with either gastric or metaplastic epithelium. Some authors have indicated a possible link between gastritis cystica profunda and carcinoma (Quizilbash, 1975). Fundic gland cysts usually present as small, multiple polyps in the body of the stomach, and are regarded as hamartomas (Sipponen et al, 1983)

(Fig. 74). They have no malignant potential but have been
described in patients with adenomatosis (familial polyposis coli).

DUODENUM AND SMALL INTESTINE

A. Adenoma (including those in adenomatosis) (Figs. 75–77)

Although uncommon, this is the usual form in which epithelial
dysplasia is represented in the small intestine. Adenomas may
occur as single or multiple lesions. A site of predilection is the
ampulla of Vater. Solitary adenomas may be tubular, but more
frequently tubulovillous or villous, and exhibit all grades of
dysplasia (Figs. 75 and 76). They differ little from their counter-
parts in the colorectum. The incidence of multiple adenomas in
familial adenomatosis coli is at least 50%, especially in association
with Gardner's syndrome, but most are small and show only a mild
degree of dysplasia (Phillips, 1981) (Fig. 77). Large adenomas
with severe dysplasia occur mainly in the vicinity of the ampulla of
Vater (Jones and Nance, 1977).

B. Dysplasia in Peutz–Jeghers polyps (Figs. 78 and 79)

There is a slightly increased risk of gastrointestinal malignancy in
patients with the Peutz–Jeghers syndrome. Epithelial dysplasia has
been observed, albeit rarely in the gastric, small intestinal and
colorectal polyps, and probably represents the histogenetic link
between this lesion and carcinoma (Gibbs, 1978). Misplacement of
mucosa (sometimes associated with the formation of mucous cysts)
into the tissues of the bowel wall should not be mistaken for
carcinoma.

C. Dysplasia in Crohn's disease (Figs. 80 and 81)

The increased risk of carcinoma in this condition may be related to
the development of dysplasia, which has been observed in a
proportion of those cases in which the association was sought
(Simpson et al, 1981). The changes are diffuse, occur in flat mucosa
and vary from mild to severe.

APPENDIX

A. Adenoma (cystadenoma) (Figs. 82–88)

This is found rarely, may be tubular, tubulovillous or villous in
type, and becomes modified by the secretion of mucus to form a
mucinous cystadenoma (Figs. 84–86). The distinction from a simple mucocele may be difficult and is largely based on the presence
of dysplastic cells arranged in papillary formations rather than the
flattened epithelium typical of simple mucocele. Microadenomas
can be found in patients with familial adenomatosis coli (Bussey,
1975) (Figs. 82 and 83). Dysplasia is graded as for adenomas of the
colorectum and independently of the histological type. Rare
hyperplastic (metaplastic) polyps of the appendix have been con-

9

fused with adenomas, especially when showing an exaggerated papillary configuration (Figs. 87 and 88).

COLORECTUM

A. Adenoma (a focal lesion, pedunculated or sessile, characterized by epithelial dysplasia) (Figs. 89–100)

The majority of adenomas never become malignant. The magnitude of risk depends on a number of factors including size, number, presence of a villous component and grade of dysplasia (Muto et al, 1975). The risk is also affected by age, a family history of colorectal cancer and the existence of either a synchronous or a metachronous carcinoma. However, the most selective histological marker of increased cancer risk is severe dysplasia (Konishi and Morson, 1982).

The appearances vary according to the histologic type (tubular, tubulovillous or villous), the direction and level of differentiation of the constituent cells, and the grade of cytological atypia. With increasing dysplasia mucus secretion is reduced, though this is not invariable (Fig. 100). The cytoplasm generally stains more darkly, but conversely may be pale and eosinophilic (Fig. 100). As the nuclei increase in size, they show chromatin clumping, a prominent nucleolus and an increased mitotic rate. They also become elongated and pseudostratified, particularly if the dysplasia is accompanied by marked cellular crowding. However, this is not a prerequisite for the diagnosis of severe dysplasia. Paneth cells and endocrine cells are often present, but in small numbers and scattered haphazardly.

When dysplasia is severe but invasion of the muscularis mucosae has not occurred, the term 'carcinoma-in-situ' is appropriate. When invasion of the lamina propria has occurred, the most accurate descriptive term is 'intramucosal carcinoma'. However, intramucosal carcinoma of the colorectum, unlike the stomach, cannot metastasize★ and for this reason invasive carcinoma should only be reported when spread through the muscularis mucosae into the submucosa has been demonstrated. To prevent potential confusion the term intramucosal carcinoma is best avoided in the colon. Pseudoinvasion must be distinguished from infiltrating carcinoma (Fig. 84).

The three histological types of adenoma may each be graded as showing mild, moderate or severe dysplasia, as described for gastric dysplasia (Kozuka, 1975). A villous component contributes to the risk of malignant change, perhaps by increasing the surface area of the polyp.

1. *Tubular adenoma:* A neoplasm with branching tubules embedded in the lamina propria occupying at least 80% of the tumour. It is usually pedunculated but can be sessile or flat (Figs. 89–93).

2. *Villous adenoma:* A neoplasm of which at least 80% is composed of finger-like processes covered by epithelium that reaches down to the muscularis mucosae. It is usually sessile and may

★ In contrast to gastric and small intestinal mucosa, the colorectal mucous membrane contains no lymphatics above the muscularis mucosae (Fenoglio et al, 1973).

sometimes be flat and difficult to recognize macroscopically. The lining columnar cells frequently retain the capacity to secrete mucus (Figs. 94–96).

3. *Tubulovillous adenoma:* A neoplasm showing both tubular and villous structures. It can be sessile or pedunculated (Figs. 97 and 98).

B. Adenomatosis (familial polyposis coli) (Figs. 101–103)

This precancerous condition is characterized by a dominant inheritance, the presence of at least 100 colorectal adenomas, and the inevitable development of colorectal cancer. The adenomas are usually of the tubular variety but villous and tubulovillous types are also encountered (Bussey, 1975).

C. Dysplasia in juvenile polyps (Figs. 104–110)

In patients with multiple juvenile polyps (juvenile polyposis), the cancer risk is less than for familial adenomatosis, but significant nonetheless. The polyps are composed of tubules and cysts separated by an excess of lamina propria. The epithelium lining the tubules resembles normal colorectum. The development of dysplasia has been well documented and probably accounts for the increased cancer risk associated with this lesion when occurring in the form of multiple polyps (Sandler and Lipper, 1981). Inflammation due to retained mucin and infection may promote reactive changes in the epithelium that could mimic dysplasia.

D. Dysplasia in hyperplastic (metaplastic) polyps
(Figs. 111–113)

Some reports have suggested that large, multiple hyperplastic polyps may be associated with an increased, albeit slight, risk of dysplasia (Fig. 113) and even malignant change (Sumner et al, 1981). Hyperplastic polyps show lengthened crypts with a tendency to serration and cystic dilatation. There is an increase in the ratio of columnar cells to goblet cells. The cells of the lower third of the crypt are hyperplastic. The epithelium of the deep portion of the crypts sometimes shows proliferative activity which may simulate dysplasia (Figs. 111 and 112). This, however, does not extend superficially as in an adenoma. Furthermore, the deep crypts of hyperplastic polyps frequently impinge on the muscularis mucosae, which itself may be fragmented. Rarely, hyperplastic polyps can proliferate deep in the mucosa in a manner similar to the so-called 'inverted papillomas' at other sites.

E. Dysplasia in ulcerative colitis (Figs. 114–132)

An increased risk of developing colorectal cancer is seen in patients who have extensive colitis and a history of disease for ten years (Butt and Morson, 1981). Within this group, severe or high grade dysplasia is the most selective marker of cancer risk. Only a very small proportion of all patients with ulcerative colitis will require close colonoscopic surveillance. The histologic picture of dysplasia

11

in ulcerative colitis tends to be varied, in a manner analogous to the epithelial alterations encountered in chronic gastritis.

Specimens may be categorized as negative, indefinite or positive for dysplasia (Riddell et al, 1983):

1. *Negative:* This implies that dysplasia is not seen. However, the distinction between reactive or reparative change and dysplasia may be difficult. Epithelium showing reactive changes reveals active inflammation, with infiltration by neutrophils. The nuclei may be enlarged with variation of size and shape and the nucleoli may be prominent and eosinophilic. However, the nuclei also tend to be vesicular with a delicate nuclear membrane rather than hyperchromatic, and the actual number of nuclei per unit area is not obviously increased. The colonoscopic findings and clinical setting will provide contributory evidence (Figs. 114–116).

2. *Indefinite:* There are two indications for the use of this category. Cytological atypia in the presence of active inflammation may occasionally be too marked to permit a negative report. In this situation, an indefinite report implies the need for further biopsies to assess the effects of time and therapy. Secondly, various types of epithelial growth pattern may be observed whose significance is, at present, unknown. These patterns have a counterpart in chronic atrophic gastritis and particularly within the entity of incomplete intestinal metaplasia. They include:

(i) Incomplete maturation (basal cell hyperplasia): Goblet cells are reduced in number or lacking altogether. The glands are lined by immature columnar cells with eosinophilic cytoplasm, round or oval basal nuclei, and sometimes apical mucin droplets. The distinction from regenerative change may be difficult (Figs. 127 and 128).

(ii) Hyperplastic (metaplastic) growth pattern: Resembles the hyperplastic polyp of the colorectum (Figs. 129 and 130).

(iii) Follicular proctitis (colitis): The epithelium overlying the numerous lymphoid aggregates shows the regenerative-type changes described above (Fig. 115).

It must be stressed that within these three patterns the cytological changes may be sufficient to permit a positive diagnosis of dysplasia.

3. *Positive:* Adenomatous dysplasia is the most usual and well known type. Macroscopically the mucosa appears velvety or nodular. Microscopically a low villous pattern is seen more frequently than a tubular type of proliferation. The lining epithelium is similar to that of colorectal adenomas and the dysplasia may be graded mild, moderate or severe. Alternatively, the terms 'low grade' and 'high grade' may be used, the latter being virtually synonymous with moderate and severe dysplasia. Dysplasia may also occur in one of the epithelial growth patterns outlined in the 'indefinite' category. These tend to present in a flat mucosa and the commonest is basal cell proliferation (see above). Additional forms are encountered, albeit rarely, including clear cell dysplasia, pancellular dysplasia (affecting all cell lines including Paneth cells and endocrine cells) and in-situ carcinoma (essentially intramucosal carcinoma). There are at present no definite guidelines for grading these non-adenomatous types of dysplasia (Riddell, 1976). Mis-

placement of glands within the submucosa (e.g. in colitis cystica profunda) must be distinguished from infiltrating carcinoma (Riddell, 1976).

Discrete adenomas may occasionally arise in colitic mucosa. It is important to ensure that dysplasia does not extend into the adjacent flat mucosa.

F. Dysplasia in Crohn's disease

The risk of developing colorectal cancer in Crohn's disease is increased, albeit slightly. Dysplasia has been observed in the mucosa adjacent to carcinoma in Crohn's disease (Craft et al, 1981). The discovery of dysplasia in biopsies may be of value for individual patients, but screening patients for dysplasia in Crohn's disease is unlikely to be an effective measure in cancer prevention (Butt and Morson, 1981). Misplaced glands within the submucosa may be confused with infiltrating carcinoma.

G. Dysplasia in schistosomiasis japonica

The chronic colitis of schistosomiasis japonica is complicated by epithelial dysplasia and carcinoma in a manner analogous to chronic ulcerative colitis (Ming-Chai et al, 1980). Screening may therefore be appropriate in those regions of Asia where this infestation is endemic.

H. Dysplasia following ureterosigmoidostomy (Fig. 133)

Polypoid tumours may complicate implantation of ureters into the sigmoid colon (or small intestine). These resemble inflammatory or juvenile polyps, but may show areas of dysplasia and malignant change (Ansell and Vellacott, 1980).

I. Transitional mucosa (Figs. 134–137)

This refers to altered epithelium bordering colorectal cancers (Filipe and Branfoot, 1976). The mucosa is thickened and composed of branched crypts lined by tall goblet cells (Fig. 136). The latter secrete sialomucin but, unlike normal colorectal mucosa, little or no sulphomucin (Figs. 135 and 137). Compressed inconspicuously between the goblet cells are immature intermediate cells secreting small amounts of apical sulphomucin (Fig.137). Similar, but not necessarily identical, changes have been observed in a number of non-cancerous settings (Isaacson and Attwood, 1979). It is unclear whether transitional mucosa is precancerous or reactive.

J. Lesions simulating dysplasia

Reactive and regenerative changes may mimic dysplasia as described at other sites. This is especially the case in ulcerative colitis (Fig. 115), but is not otherwise as common in the colon as in the stomach. Pseudoinvasion or epithelial misplacement occurs in a variety of conditions (see above) and must be distinguished from

13

infiltrating carcinoma. Other conditions associated with epithelial misplacement include the solitary ulcer syndrome, mucosal prolapse and endometriosis. Dysplasia following irradiation requires care in interpretation (see Oesophagus: D.3).

ANAL CANAL

The epithelium above the dentate line is of rectal type except for the narrow transitional (junctional, cloacogenic) zone. The epithelium lining the latter varies with age as well as pathological conditions. Rectal mucosa, stratified columnar epithelium, transitional epithelium (resembling that of the urinary tract), and squamous epithelium may all be represented within this complex area. A squamous mucous membrane is seen below the dentate line, devoid of pilosebaceous follicles and sweat glands. This extends to the anal margin which is lined by skin.

A. Dysplasia and carcinoma-in-situ (Figs. 138–140)

The microscopic appearances are similar to the analogous lesions of the oesophagus and cervix. The epithelium is thickened and there is proliferation of atypical basal cells showing enlarged, hyperchromatic nuclei and numerous mitoses. With increasing dysplasia the proportion of the epithelium occupied by these cells also increases. Ultimately a stage of carcinoma-in-situ is reached when atypical basal cells extend up to the surface.

These lesions are seen more frequently in the transitional mucosa above the dentate line than in the squamous mucous membrane of the lower anal canal. The changes are sometimes observed when haemorrhoids are examined histologically.

B. Dysplasia in leukoplakia

The lower portion of prolapsing internal haemorrhoids may appear white due to squamous metaplasia and hyperkeratosis in the transitional zone. This has no precancerous significance. Dysplasia and carcinoma-in-situ may present as a white plaque.

ANAL MARGIN

A. Dysplasia (Figs. 141 and 142)

Dysplasia and carcinoma-in-situ may occur in the epithelium of the anal margin as well as in the condylomatous lesions described below and in the rare leukoplakias that may be found at this site. The appearances are similar to those of dysplasia in the anal canal.

B. Condyloma acuminatum (viral wart) (Figs. 143–146)

This may be regarded as part of a spectrum of squamous cell tumours which include not only the common, benign and easily curable lesions but also the locally aggressive giant condylomas. Malignant change has been reported but is rare. The lesions typically show a papillary acanthosis, parakeratosis, vacuolation of cells in the upper epidermis, and underlying chronic inflammation.

Giant condyloma (verrucous carcinoma) is a very large, histologically bland yet clinically aggressive squamous neoplasm occurring in the perianal region and genitalia (Dawson et al, 1965) (Figs. 145 and 146). Biologically similar lesions occur in the sole of the foot (carcinoma cuniculatum), in the mouth, and in the upper respiratory tract (verrucous carcinoma). This is not a precancerous lesion; it is mentioned here because of its deceptively innocuous histologic appearance.

C. Paget's disease (Fig. 147)

This is characterized by the presence within the epidermis of large, pale, sialomucin-filled cells. The vesicular nucleus is displaced to one side, giving a signet-ring appearance. The lesion may be found in isolation or in association with intraduct or infiltrating carcinoma of underlying glands. Unlike Paget's disease of the breast, the intraductal phase tends to be of long duration. Some might consider Paget's disease to be a cancerous rather than a precancerous lesion (Linder and Myers, 1970).

D. Bowen's disease (Figs. 141, 142, 148 and 149)

This occurs only rarely in the perianal region. Its features are similar to its occurrence at other sites. Bowenoid papulosis resembles Bowen's disease histologically, but not clinically. It presents in young adults with multiple reddish papules in the perianal area, vulva or penis. In spite of its disturbing histology, including enlarged, vacuolated cells with atypical nuclei (Figs. 148 and 149), conservative therapy appears to eradicate the lesion (Wade et al, 1978).

References

Andreasen J. O. (1968) Oral lichen planus. II. A histologic evaluation of ninety-seven cases. *Oral Surgery* 25: 158–166.

Ansell I. D. & Vellacott K. D. (1980) Colonic polyps complicating ureterosigmoidostomy. *Histopathology* 4: 429–436.

Barge J., Molas G., Maillard J. N., Fekete F., Bogolometz W. W. & Potet F. (1981) Superficial oesophageal carcinoma: an oesophageal counterpart of early gastric cancer. *Histopathology* 5: 499–510.

Berenson M. M., Herbst J. J. & Freston J. W. (1974) Enzyme and ultrastructural characteristics of esophageal columnar epithelium. *American Journal of Digestive Diseases* 19: 895–907.

Berenson M. M., Riddell R. G., Skinner D. B. & Freston J. W. (1978) Malignant transformation of oesophageal columnar epithelium. *Cancer* 41: 554–561.

Berthrong M. & Fajardo L. F. (1981) Radiation injury in surgical pathology, part II: alimentary tract. *American Journal of Surgical Pathology* 5: 153–178.

Bussey H. J. R. (1975) *Familial Polyposis Coli*. Baltimore: Johns Hopkins University Press.

Butt J. H. & Morson B. C. (1981) Dysplasia and cancer in inflammatory bowel disease. *Gastroenterology* 80: 865–868.

Craft C. F., Mendelsohn G., Cooper H. S. & Yardley J. H. (1981) Colonic 'Precancer' in Crohn's disease. *Gastroenterology* 80: 578–584.

Cuello C., Correa P., Zarama G., López J., Murray J. & Gordillo G. (1979) Histopathology of gastric dysplasia. *American Journal of Surgical Pathology* 3: 491–500.

Dawson D. F., Duckworth J. J., Bernhardt H. & Young J. M. (1965) Giant condyloma and verrucous carcinoma of the genital area. *Archives of Pathology* 79: 225–231.

Elster K. (1976) Histological classification of gastric polyps. In Morson B. C. (ed.): *Current Topics in Pathology*, vol 63, pp. 77–99. Berlin: Springer-Verlag.

Fenoglio C. M., Kaye G. I. & Lane N. (1973) Distribution of human colonic lymphatics in normal, hyperplastic and adenomatous tissue. *Gastroenterology* 64: 51–66.

Filipe M. I. & Branfoot A. C. (1976) Mucin histochemistry of the colon. In Morson B. C. (ed.): *Current Topics in Pathology*, vol. 63, pp. 143–178. Berlin: Springer-Verlag.

Filipe M. I. & Lake B. D. (1983) *Histochemistry in Pathology*. Edinburgh: Churchill Livingstone.

Franzin G. & Novelli P. (1981) Gastritis cystica profunda. *Histopathology* 5: 535–547.

Gibbs N. M. (1978) Juvenile and Peutz–Jeghers polyps. In Morson B. C. (ed.): *The Pathogenesis of Colorectal Cancer*, pp. 21–32. (Major Problems in Pathology vol. 10). Philadelphia: W. B. Saunders.

Isaacson P. & Attwood P. R. A. (1979) Failure to demonstrate specificity of the morphological and histochemical changes adjacent to colonic carcinoma (transitional mucosa). *Journal of Clinical Pathology* 32: 214–218.

Jass J. R. (1980) Role of intestinal metaplasia in the histogenesis of gastric carcinoma. *Journal of Clinical Pathology* 33: 801–810.

Jass J. R. (1981) Mucin histochemistry of the columnar epithelium of the oesophagus. *Journal of Clinical Pathology* 34: 866–870.

Jass J. R. (1983) A classification of gastric dysplasia. *Histopathology* 7: 181–193.

Jones T. R. & Nance F. C. (1977) Periampullary malignancy in Gardner's syndrome. *Annals of Surgery* 185: 565–573.

Kamiya T., Morishita T., Asakura H., Miura S., Munakata Y. & Tsuchiya M. (1981) Histoclinical long-standing follow-up study of hyperplastic polyps of the stomach. *American Journal of Gastroenterology* 75: 275–281.

Konishi F. & Morson B. C. (1982) Pathology of colorectal adenomas: a colonoscopic survey. *Journal of Clinical Pathology* 35: 830–841.

Kozuka S. (1975) Premalignancy of the mucosal polyp in the large intestine. I. Histologic gradation on the basis of epithelial pseudo-stratification and glandular branching. *Diseases of the Colon and Rectum* 18: 483–493.

Linder J. H. & Myers R. T. (1970) Perianal Paget's disease. *American Surgeon* 36: 342–345.

Mandard A. M., Tourneaux J., Gignouz M., Blanc L., Segol P., & Mandard J. C. (1980) In situ carcinoma of the oesophagus. Macroscopic study with particular reference to the Lugol test. *Endoscopy* 12: 51–57.

McKay J. S. & Day D. W. (1983) Herpes simplex oesophagitis. *Histopathology* 7: 409–420.

Ming S-C. (1977) The classification and significance of gastric polyps. In Yardley J. H., Morson B. C. & Abell M. R. (eds.): *The Gastrointestinal Tract*, pp. 149–175. (IAP Monograph.) Baltimore: Williams & Wilkins.

Ming-Chai C., Chi-Yuan C., Pei-Yu C. & Jen-Chun H. (1980) Evolution of colorectal cancer in schistosomiasis: transitional changes adjacent to large intestinal carcinoma in colectomy specimens. *Cancer* 46: 1661–1675.

Morson B. C., Sobin L. H., Grundmann E., Johansen A., Nagayo T. & Serck-Hannsen A. (1980) Precancerous conditions and epithelial dysplasia of the stomach. *Journal of Clinical Pathology* 33: 231–240.

Muñoz N., Crespi M., Grassi A., Qing W. G., Qiong S. & Cai L. Z. (1982) Precursor lesions of oesophageal cancer in high-risk populations in Iran and China. *Lancet* i: 876–879.

Muto T., Bussey H. J. R. & Morson B. C. (1975) The evolution of cancer of the colon and rectum. *Cancer* 36: 2251–2270.

Nagayo T. (1971) Histological diagnosis of biopsied gastric mucosa with special reference to that of borderline lesions. *Gann Monograph on Cancer Research* 11: 245–256.

Nagayo T. (1981) Dysplasia of the gastric mucosa and its relation to the precancerous state. *Gann* 72: 813–823.

O'Brien C. J., Saverymuttu S., Hodgson H. J. F. & Evans D. J. (1983) Coeliac disease, adenocarcinoma of jejunum and in-situ squamous carcinoma of the oesophagus. *Journal of Clinical Pathology* 36: 62–67.

Oehlert W., Keller P., Henke M. & Straube M. (1979) Gastric mucosal dysplasias: what is their clinical significance? *Frontiers of Gastrointestinal Research* 4: 173–182.

Ozzello L., Savary M. & Roethlisberger B. (1977) Columnar mucosa of the distal oesophagus in patients with gastroesophageal reflux. In Sommers S. C. & Rosen P. P. (eds.): *Pathology Annual* vol. 12, pp. 41–86. New York: Appleton-Century-Crofts.

Paull A., Trier J. S., Dalton M. D., Camp R. C., Loeb P. & Goyal R. K. (1976) The histologic spectrum of Barrett's esophagus. *New England Journal of Medicine* 295: 476–480.

References

Phillips L. G. (1981) Polyposis and carcinoma of the small bowel and familial colonic polyposis. *Diseases of the Colon and Rectum* 24: 478–481.

Quizilbash A. H. (1975) Gastritis cystica and carcinoma arising in old gastrojejunostomy stomach. *Canadian Medical Association Journal* 112: 1432–1433.

Riddell R. H. (1976) The precarcinomatous phase of ulcerative colitis. In Morson B. C. (ed.): *Pathology of the Gastrointestinal Tract*, pp. 179–219. (Current Topics in Pathology, vol. 63.) Berlin: Springer-Verlag.

Riddell R. H., Goldman H., Ransohoff D. F., Appelman H. D., Fenoglio C. M., Haggitt R. C., Åhren C., Correa P., Hamilton S. R., Morson B. C., Sommers S. C. & Yardley J. H. (1983) Dysplasia in inflammatory bowel disease. Standardised classification with provisional clinical applications. *Human Pathology* 14: 931–969.

Sandler R. S. & Lipper S. (1981) Multiple adenomas in juvenile polyposis. *American Journal of Gastroenterology* 75: 361–366.

Segura D. I. & Montero C. (1983) Histochemical characterisation of different types of intestinal metaplasia in gastric mucosa. *Cancer* 52: 498–503.

Simpson S., Traube J. & Riddell R. H. (1981) The histologic appearance of dysplasia (precancerous change) in Crohn's disease of the small and large intestine. *Gastroenterology* 81: 492–501.

Sipponen P., Seppälä K., Varis K., Hjelt L., Ihamaki T., Kekki M. & Siurala M. (1980) Intestinal metaplasia with colonic-type sulphomucins in the gastric mucosa; its association with gastric carcinoma. *Acta Pathologica et Microbiologica Scandinavica* A88: 217–224.

Sipponen P., Laxén F. & Seppälä K. (1983) Cystic 'hamartomatous' gastric polyps: a disorder of oxyntic glands. *Histopathology* 7: 729–737.

Sugano H., Nakamura K. & Takagi K. (1971) An atypical epithelium of the stomach. *Gann Monograph on Cancer Research* 11: 257–269.

Sumner H. W., Wasserman N. F., McClain C. J. (1981) Giant hyperplastic polyposis of the colon. *Digestive Diseases and Sciences* 26: 85–89.

Tomasulo J. (1971) Gastric polyps: histologic types and their relationship to gastric carcinoma. *Cancer* 27: 1346–1355.

Trier J. S. (1970) Morphology of the epithelium of the distal oesophagus in patients with mid-oesophageal peptic stricture. *Gastroenterology* 58: 444–461.

Trier J. S. & Curtis R. L. (1983) Barrett's oesophagus. In Jerzy-Glass G. B. & Sherlock P. (eds.): *Progress in Gastroenterology*, vol. 4, pp. 231–252. New York: Grune & Stratton.

Ushigome S., Spjut H. J. & Noon G. P. (1967) Extensive dysplasia and carcinoma-in-situ of oesophageal epithelium. *Cancer* 20: 1023–1029.

Wade T. R., Kopf A. W. & Ackerman A. B. (1978) Bowenoid papulosis of the penis. *Cancer* 42: 1890–1903.

List of Figures

The original 35 mm transparencies have been enlarged by a factor of 4 for printed page reproduction. The magnification factor quoted in the legend refers to the printed photograph. When a higher power view is shown it will always follow immediately after the low power view.

List of Figures

Fig. 1
*Normal stratified
squamous epithelium,
oesophagus*

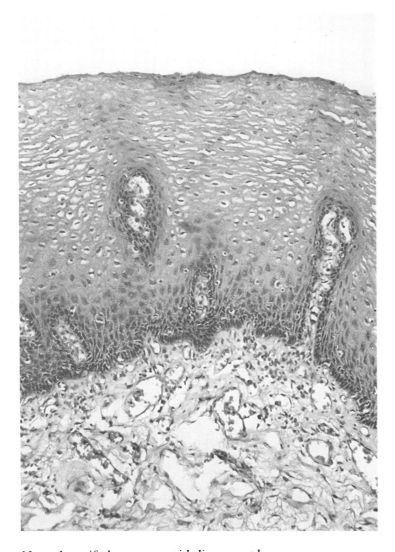

Normal stratified squamous epithelium, oesophagus

The non-keratinized, squamous epithelium, shows no abnormal features.

H&E. ×250.

Fig. 2
Chronic oesophagitis

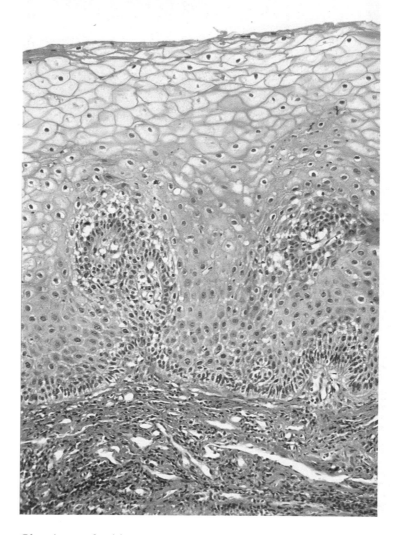

Chronic oesophagitis

There is acanthosis, clear cell change and a heavy chronic inflammatory infiltrate within the submucosa. Dysplasia is not present.

H&E. ×160.

Fig. 3
*Chronic oesophagitis
with atrophy*

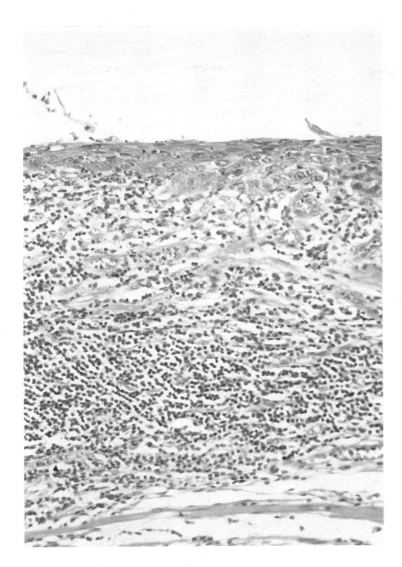

Chronic oesophagitis with atrophy

The epithelium is atrophic and shows no evidence of dysplasia. The submucosa is heavily infiltrated by chronic inflammatory cells.

H&E. ×250.

Fig. 4
*Chronic oesophagitis
due to lichen planus*

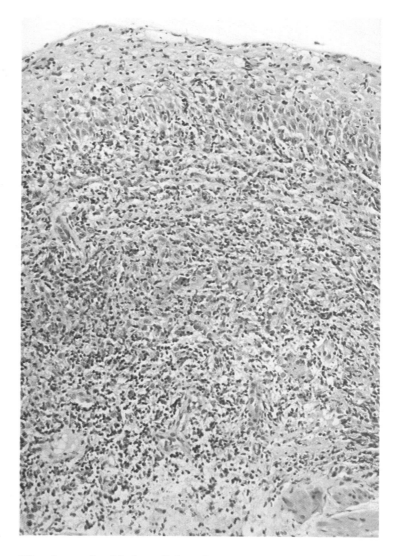

Chronic oesophagitis due to lichen planus

A dense, band-like infiltrate of chronic inflammatory cells (mainly lymphocytes but also plasma cells) is pressed up against an atrophic epithelium. (This may on other occasions be thickened and hyperkeratotic.) Diagnosis will be facilitated by the presence of oral or cutaneous involvement (see Fig. 5).

H&E. ×160.

Fig. 5
*Chronic oesophagitis
due to lichen planus*

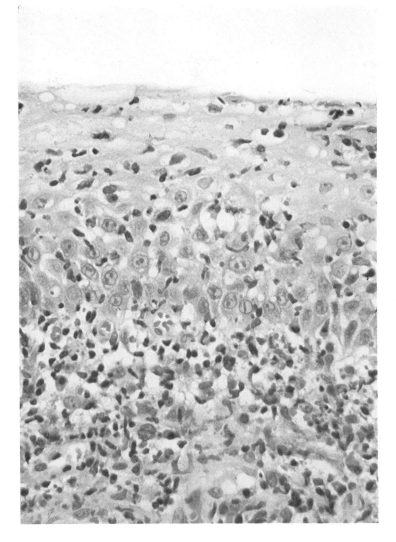

Chronic oesophagitis due to lichen planus

The epithelium is infiltrated by convoluted lymphocytes and the interface between epithelium and lamina propria has become blurred.

H&E. ×400.

Fig. 6
*Mild dysplasia,
oesophagus*

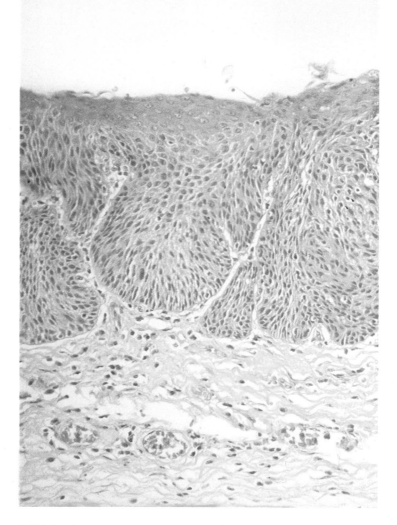

Mild dysplasia, oesophagus

Atypical basal cells with enlarged, pleomorphic nuclei occupy the lower third of the epithelium. There is cytoplasmic maturation and a lack of significant cytological atypia above this level.

H&E. ×250.

Fig. 7
*Moderate dysplasia,
oesophagus*

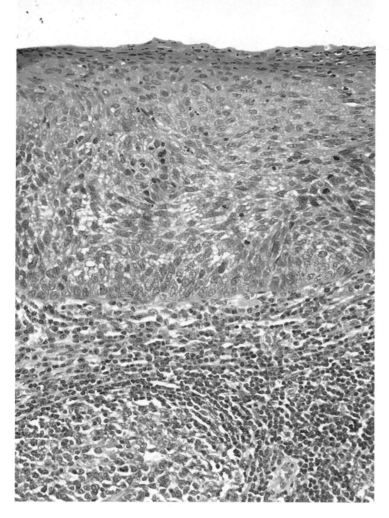

Moderate dysplasia, oesophagus

The proliferation of atypical basal cells is accompanied by aberrant
cytoplasmic maturation with hyperparakeratosis. The lesion
would have appeared as a white plaque on endoscopy.

H&E. ×250.

Fig. 8
*Severe dysplasia,
oesophagus*

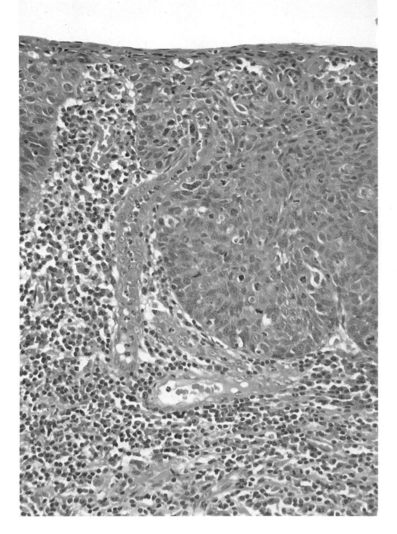

Severe dysplasia, oesophagus

The neoplastic proliferation has resulted in vertical compression of
the underlying stroma. Congested vessels come into close contact
with the mucosal surface at these points. There is hyperparakeratosis. The lesion would have appeared as a white plaque
with red punctuation on endoscopy.

H&E. ×250.

Fig. 9
Severe dysplasia,
oesophagus

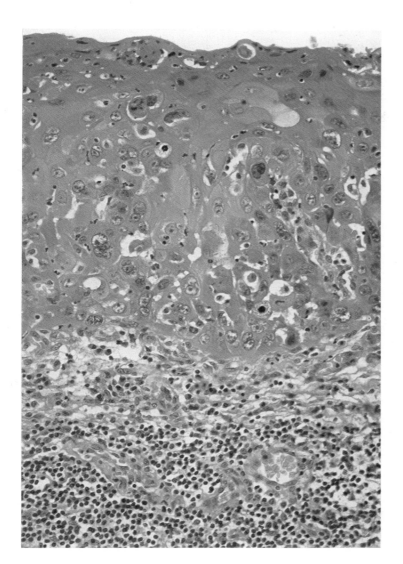

Severe dysplasia, oesophagus

The appearances contrast with those of Fig. 8 in that the dysplastic cells show an abundant, deeply eosinophilic cytoplasm. There is loss of cellular cohesion and individual cell keratinization. The nuclei are enlarged, pleomorphic and contain a prominent nucleolus. Mitoses (some atypical) are numerous.

H&E. ×250.

Fig. 10
*Indefinite change in
chronic atrophic
oesophagitis*

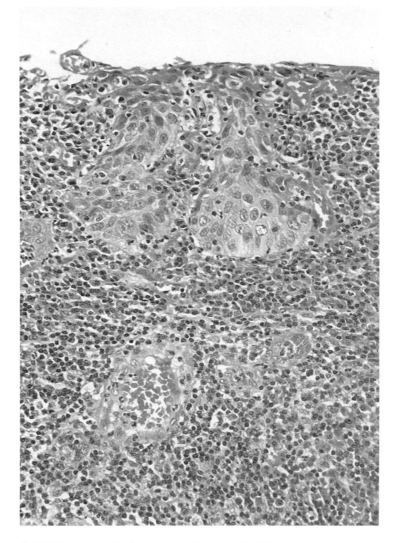

Indefinite change in chronic atrophic oesophagitis

The nuclei are enlarged but show a delicate nuclear membrane and little hyperchromatism. It is not possible to make a certain distinction between neoplastic and severe inflammatory change on this field alone. However, severe dysplasia was present in the same section.

H&E. ×250.

Fig. 11
*Severe dysplasia in
chronic atrophic
oesophagitis*

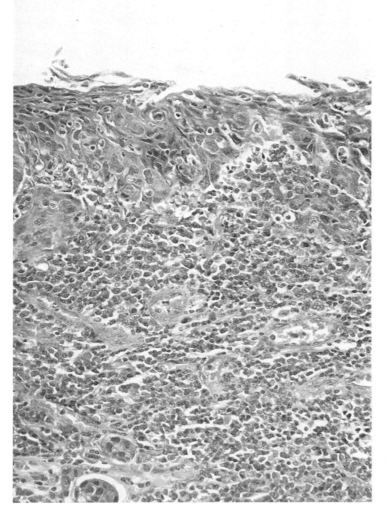

Severe dysplasia in chronic atrophic oesophagitis

Irregular tongues of neoplastic epithelium dip into an intensely
inflamed submucosa. The nuclei show marked pleomorphism and
hyperchromatism. Submucosal lymphatics show carcinomatous
infiltration.

H&E. ×250.

Fig. 12
*Dysplasia and early
oesophageal carcinoma*

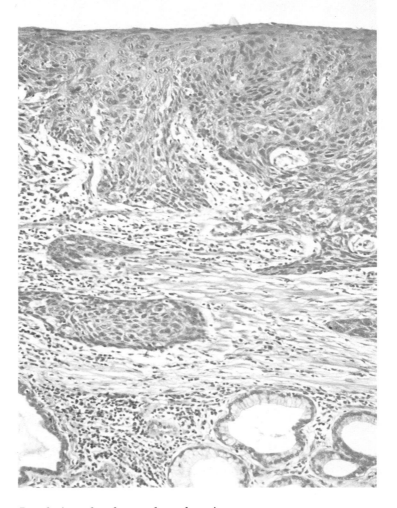

Dysplasia and early oesophageal carcinoma

Tongues of squamous cell carcinoma invade the muscularis mucosae. Atrophic submucosal glands occupy the lower field.

H&E. ×160.

Fig. 13
Normal oesophagus,
glycogen

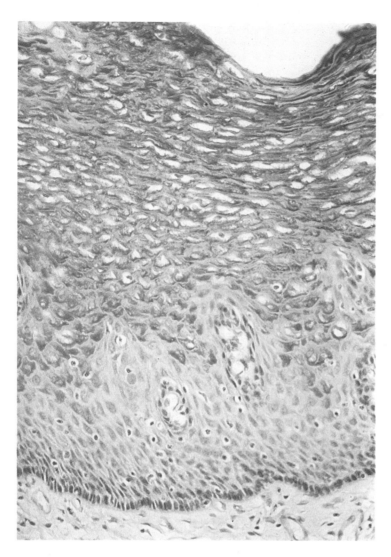

Normal oesophagus, glycogen

Normal maturation is accompanied by the intracellular accumulation of glycogen.

PAS. ×250.

Fig. 14
Moderate dysplasia and glycogen, oesophagus

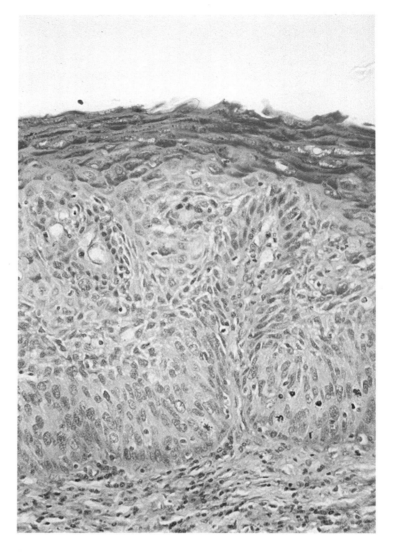

Moderate dysplasia and glycogen, oesophagus

In spite of the proliferation of atypical basal cells, superficial maturation is accompanied by glycogenation. Iodine application during endoscopy would give a positive result and therefore not detect the underlying neoplastic change.

PAS. ×250.

Fig. 15
*Severe dysplasia and
glycogen, oesophagus*

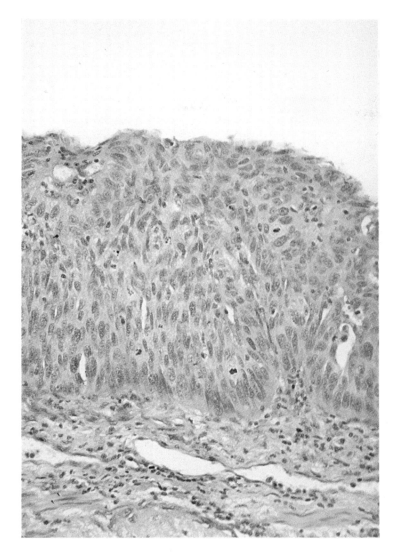

Severe dysplasia and glycogen, oesophagus

Only when the entire epithelium is replaced by atypical basal cells
(showing no maturation) will glycogen be absent.

PAS. ×250.

Fig. 16
Barrett's oesophagus,
cardiac type

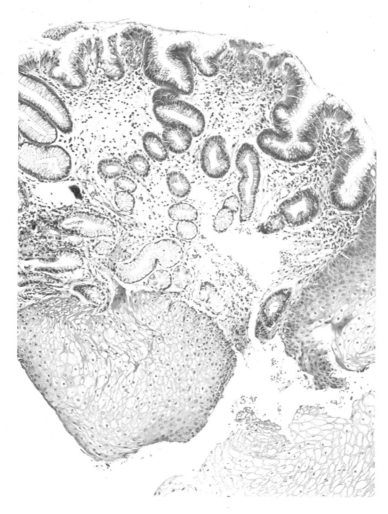

Barrett's oesophagus, cardiac type

Atrophic cardiac type mucosa adjoins squamous epithelium.
H&E. ×100.

Fig. 17
*Barrett's oesophagus,
fundic type*

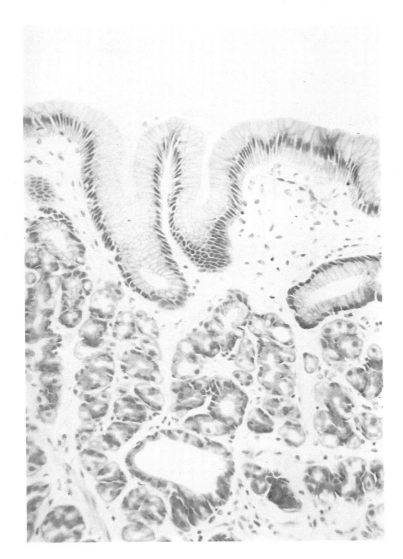

Barrett's oesophagus, fundic type
Parietal cells are readily observed.
H&E. ×250.

Fig. 18
Barrett's oesophagus,
specialized type

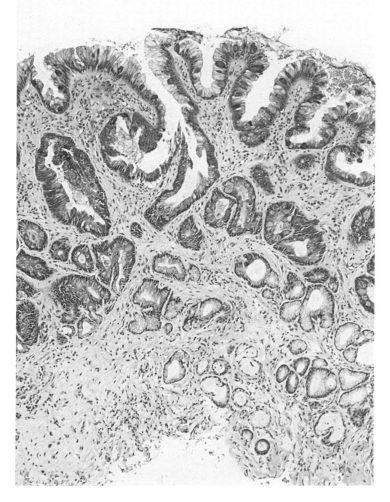

Barrett's oesophagus, specialized type

The mucosa shows atrophy, architectural irregularity (including villosity) and increased fibrosis of the lamina propria. The appearances indicate post-inflammatory regeneration (see Fig. 19).

H&E. ×100.

Fig. 19
*Barrett's oesophagus,
specialized type*

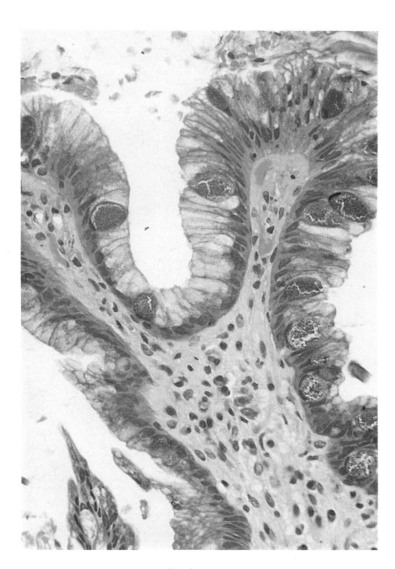

Barrett's oesophagus, specialized type

The villosities are lined by goblet cells secreting acid mucins (basophilic with Ehrlich's haematoxylin) and columnar mucous cells. (Mature intestinal-type enterocytes are rarely observed in specialized mucosa.) The appearances recall incomplete intestinal metaplasia of gastric mucosa (see Fig. 39).

H&E. ×400.

Fig. 20
*Barrett's oesophagus,
specialized type
(mucins).*

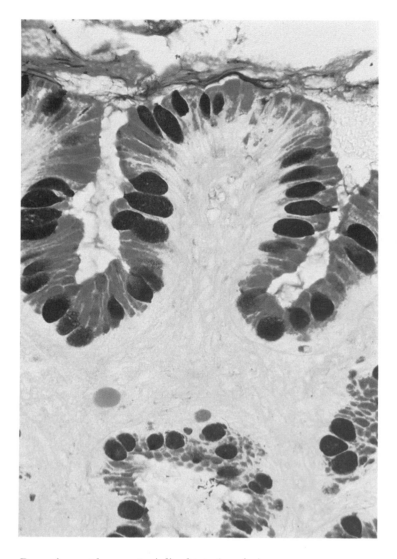

Barrett's oesophagus, specialized type (mucins).

The columnar cells (red) secrete neutral mucins, like normal gastric foveolar cells. The goblet cells (blue) secrete acid mucins.

Alcian blue/diastase PAS. ×400.

Fig. 21
*Barrett's oesophagus,
specialized type (mucins)*

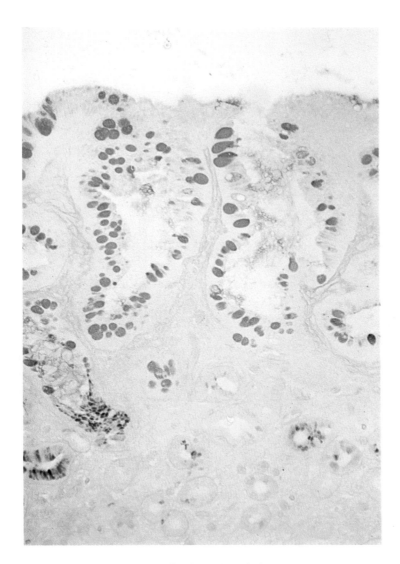

Barrett's oesophagus, specialized type (mucins).

The goblet cells secrete sialomucins (blue). The intervening crypt columnar cells produce mainly neutral mucins and are therefore virtually unstained. The underlying glands secrete sulphomucins (brown), as do some of the immature crypt base cells. Other staining patterns may be encountered. In variants associated with dysplasia and carcinoma, the crypt and surface columnar cells often secrete sulphomucins. This event will produce the appearance shown in Fig. 40.

High iron diamine/Alcian blue. ×160.

Fig. 22
*Indefinite change,
Barrett's oesophagus*

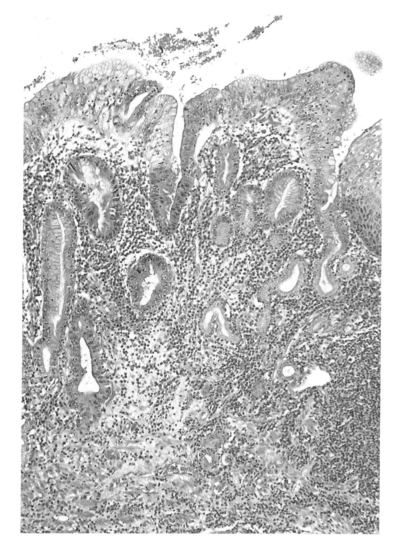

Indefinite change, Barrett's oesophagus

The cardiac type mucosa shows chronic inflammation and atrophy.
The crypts reveal regenerative change, but some are rendered
prominent by their darkly staining cytoplasm (see Fig. 23).

H&E. ×100.

Fig. 23
Indefinite change,
Barrett's oesophagus

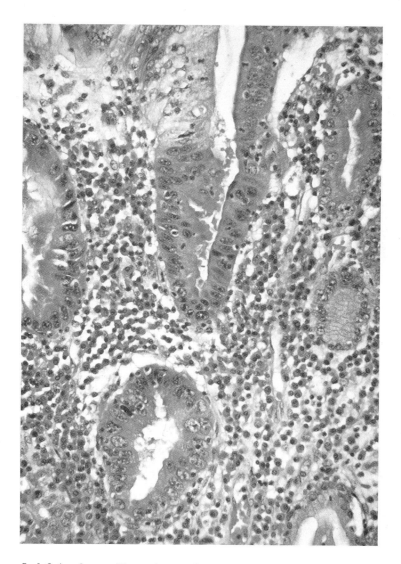

Indefinite change, Barrett's oesophagus

The nuclei are enlarged, hyperchromatic and show focal loss of polarity. Active inflammation is present and the changes cannot be designated with certainty as either neoplastic or reactive. Similar changes are observed in gastric mucosa and present similar diagnostic difficulties.

H&E. ×250.

Fig. 24
*Mild dysplasia in
Barrett's oesophagus*

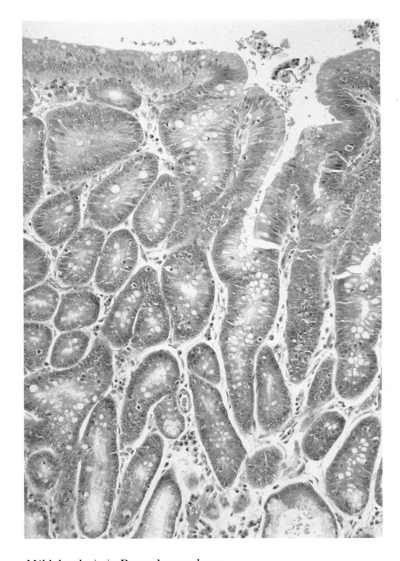

Mild dysplasia in Barrett's oesophagus

The crypts show branching and budding and are closely apposed, but not yet back to back (see Fig. 25).

H&E. ×160.

Fig. 25
*Mild dysplasia in
Barrett's oesophagus*

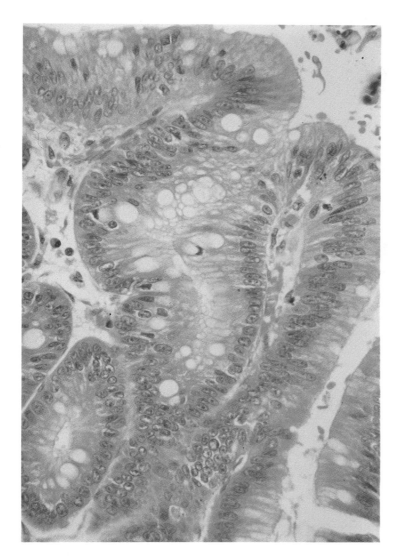

Mild dysplasia in Barrett's oesophagus

The crypts are lined by goblet cells and a population of crowded, immature mucous cells. The nuclei are slightly enlarged and vesicular, but uniform in size and shape. The appearances are of mild dysplasia in specialized mucosa.

H&E. ×400.

Fig. 26

Moderate dysplasia in Barrett's oesophagus

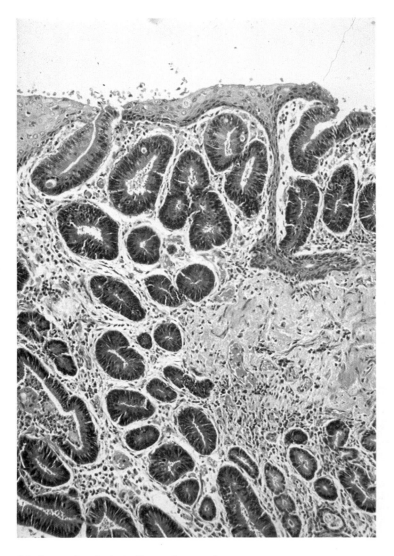

Moderate dysplasia in Barrett's oesophagus

Neoplastic tubules have proliferated below the squamous epithelium. These are lined by deeply amphophilic columnar cells and occasional goblet cells. Nuclei are enlarged, hyperchromatic and crowded with focal loss of polarity.

H&E. ×160.

Fig. 27
*Reactive change in
reflux oesophagitis
(active)*

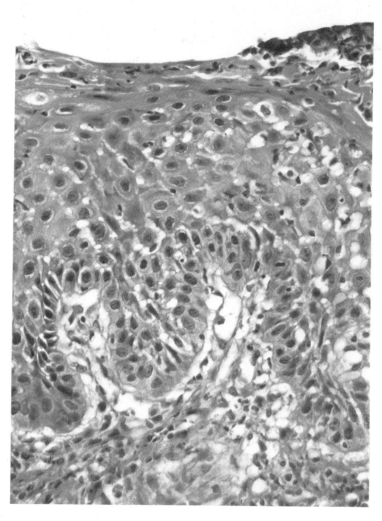

Reactive change in reflux oesophagitis (active)

The mucosa is infiltrated with acute and chronic inflammatory cells and there is intercellular oedema. The epithelial cells show a basophilic cytoplasm and an increase in the nuclear/cytoplasmic ratio. This is especially marked in the basal cell zone, where mitotic activity is increased. However, there is little pleomorphism.

H&E. ×400.

Fig. 28

Regenerative change in
reflux oesophagitis
(quiescent)

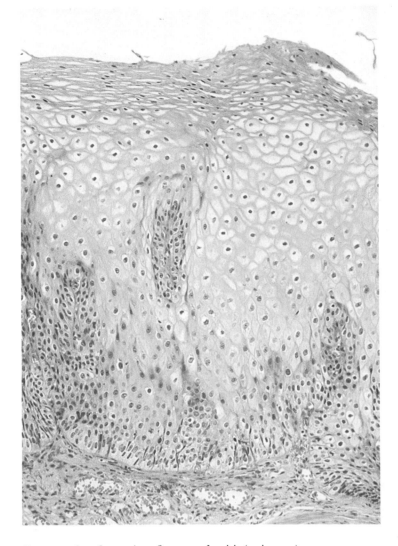

Regenerative change in reflux oesophagitis (quiescent)

The epithelium is thickened and there is vascular congestion but only mild inflammation of subepithelial tissues. The basal cell layer appears abnormally prominent. These changes may be mistaken for mild dysplasia.

H&E. ×160.

Fig. 29
Radiation change,
oesophagus

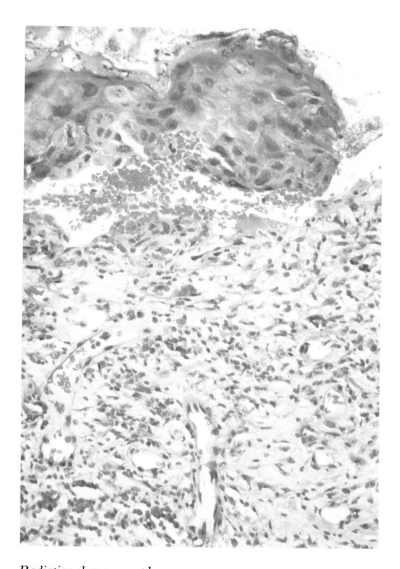

Radiation change, oesophagus

The submucosa is oedematous, mildly inflamed and includes numerous thin-walled vessels. A degenerate sheet of epithelium has separated and shows variation in nuclear size and staining. Radiation changes in both squamous epithelium and underlying tissues can simulate dysplasia and malignancy.

H&E. ×250.

Fig. 30
Superficial chronic gastritis (inactive)

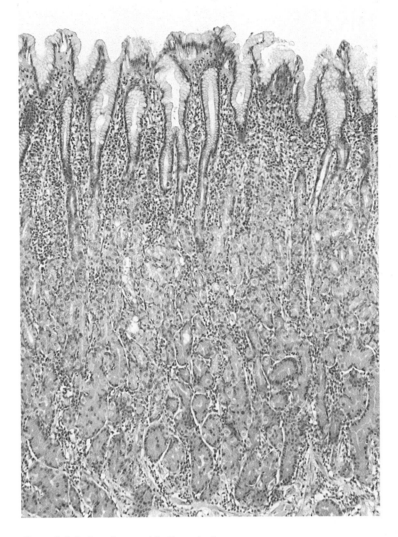

Superficial chronic gastritis (inactive)

Inflammation is confined mainly to the crypt or superficial compartment of body type mucosa. The inflammatory infiltrate includes mainly lymphocytes and plasma cells. The foveolar epithelium is unaltered.

H&E. ×160.

Fig. 31
*Chronic atrophic
gastritis (inactive)*

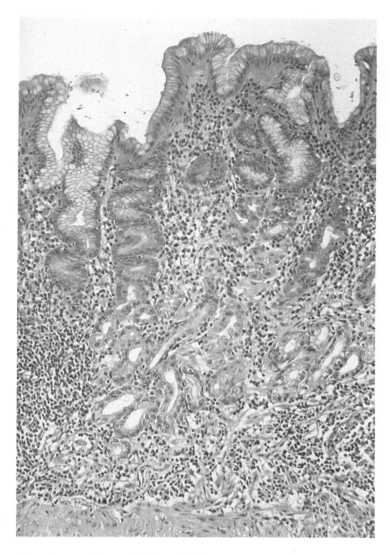

Chronic atrophic gastritis (inactive)

Inflammation extends into the deep or glandular compartment and
is accompanied by fundic gland atrophy and pyloric metaplasia.

H&E. ×160.

Fig. 32
Chronic cystic gastritis

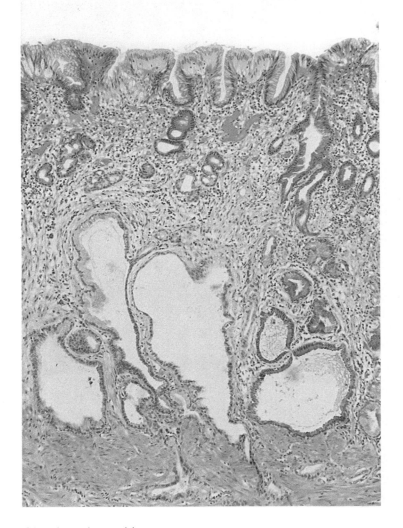

Chronic cystic gastritis

Epithelial atrophy is marked and glands are cystically dilated. Increased fibrosis of the lamina propria is conspicuous.

H&E. ×100.

Fig. 33
*Gastric atrophy with
complete intestinal
metaplasia*

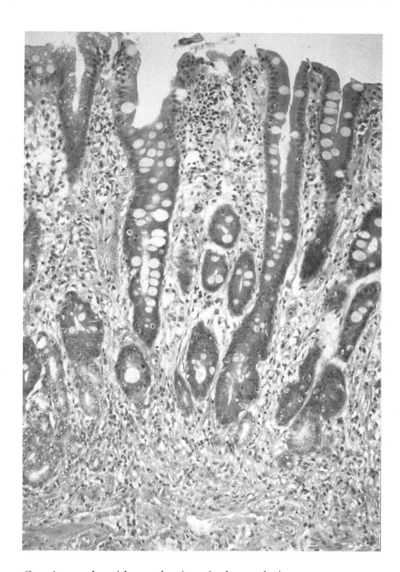

Gastric atrophy with complete intestinal metaplasia

The mucosa is thin and lined by intestinalized epithelium. This takes the form of simple, unbranched tubules. Paneth cells occupy the crypt base whereas goblet cells and eosinophilic columnar cells line the crypts and surface epithelium.

H&E. ×160.

Fig. 34
*Complete intestinal
metaplasia, stomach
(mucins)*

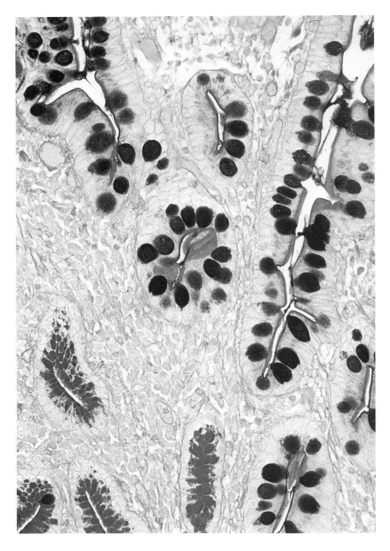

Complete intestinal metaplasia, stomach (mucins)

Absorptive cells with a well delineated brush border are bordered by goblet cells. The blue colour of the latter indicates the secretion of acid mucus. Gastric foveolar epithelium secretes neutral mucins (red).

Alcian blue/diastase PAS. ×250.

Fig. 35
*Incomplete intestinal
metaplasia, stomach*

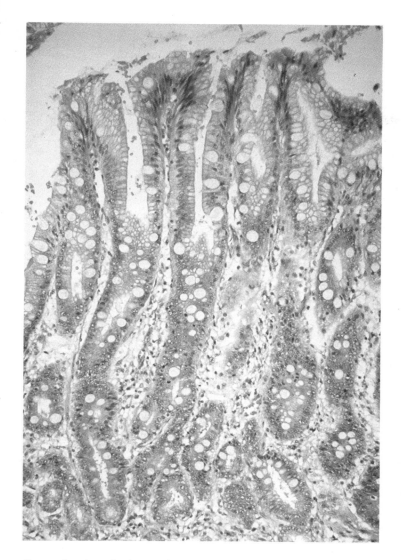

Incomplete intestinal metaplasia, stomach

The mucosa is not especially thin or atrophic and the crypts are
tortuous and branched at their bases. Paneth cells are not present
(see Fig 36).

H&E. ×160.

Fig. 36
*Incomplete intestinal
metaplasia, stomach*

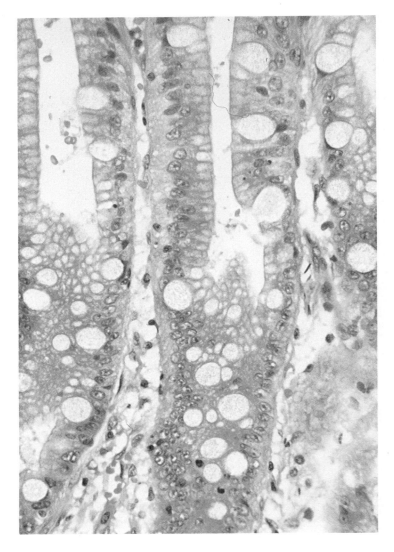

Incomplete intestinal metaplasia, stomach

The crypts are lined by goblet cells and columnar mucous cells.
The nuclei of the latter are vesicular with a prominent, though
small, nucleolus.

H&E. ×400.

Fig. 37
Complete intestinal
metaplasia, stomach

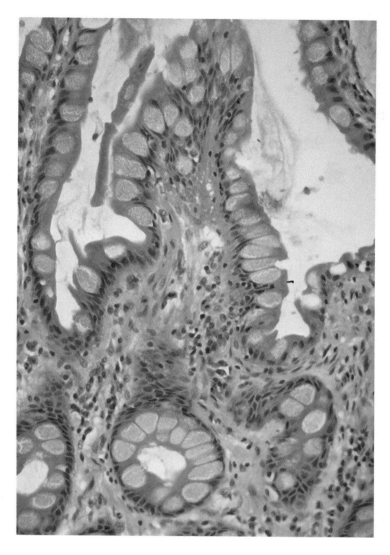

Complete intestinal metaplasia, stomach

Villi are lined by eosinophilic columnar cells and goblet cells.

H&E. ×250.

Fig. 38
Complete intestinal metaplasia, stomach (mucins)

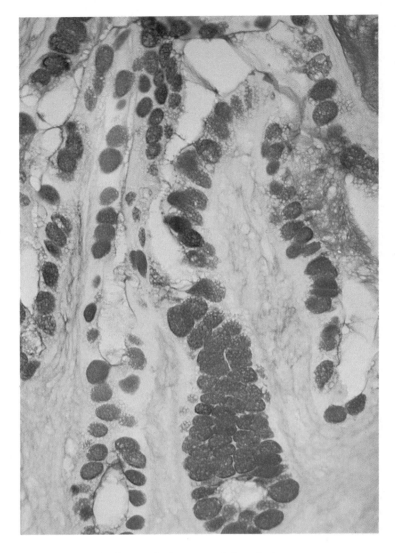

Complete intestinal metaplasia, stomach (mucins)

The goblet cells stain blue, indicating the secretion of sialomucin. The columnar cells are unstained, though their brush border is delineated.

High iron diamine/Alcian blue. ×250.

Fig. 39
*Incomplete intestinal
metaplasia, stomach*

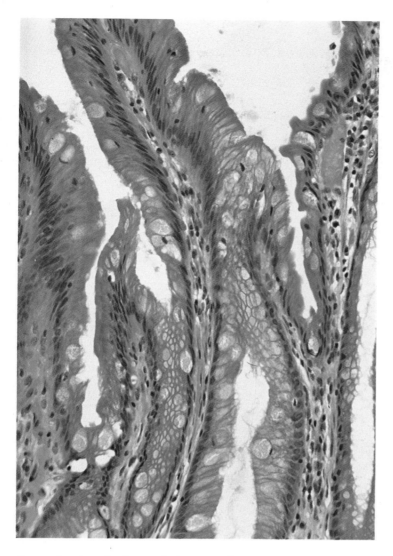

Incomplete intestinal metaplasia, stomach

The ratio of columnar cells to goblet cells is increased and the
columnar cells appear crowded and show a clear apical vesicle.

H&E. ×250.

Fig. 40

*Incomplete intestinal
metaplasia, stomach
(mucins)*

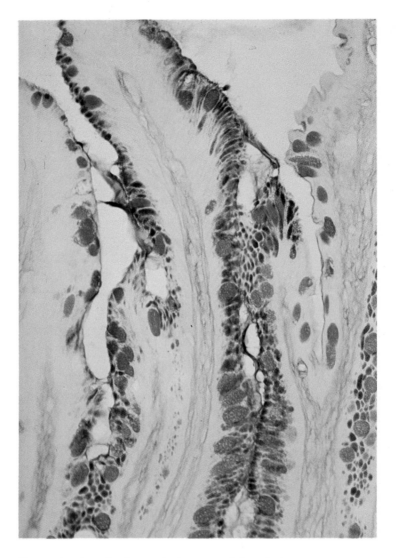

Incomplete intestinal metaplasia, stomach (mucins)

The goblet cells stain blue, indicating the secretion of
sialomucin. The columnar cells stain brown due to the
production of sulphomucin.

High iron diamine/Alcian blue. ×250.

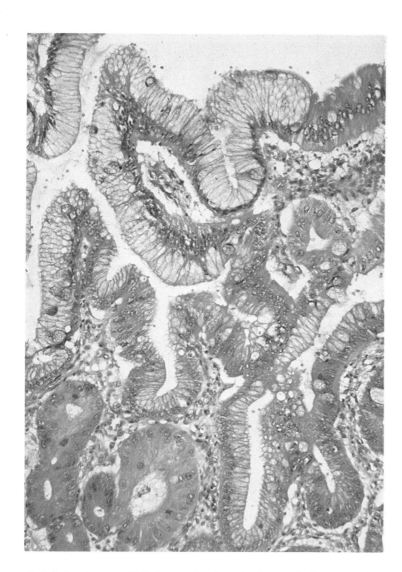

Indefinite change within incomplete intestinal metaplasia, stomach

The epithelium shows a complex arrangement with papillary processes and branched crypts. Some of the surface epithelium is lined by incomplete IM, with goblet cells bordered by tall columnar mucous cells. There are abrupt transitions to more immature-appearing epithelium in which mucus secretion is reduced. There is no active inflammation. The distinction between post-inflammatory regenerative change and mild dysplasia is not easily made. A poorly differentiated adenocarcinoma was present in the same specimen (not shown).

H&E. ×160.

Fig. 42
*Moderate dysplasia in
intestinal metaplasia,
stomach*

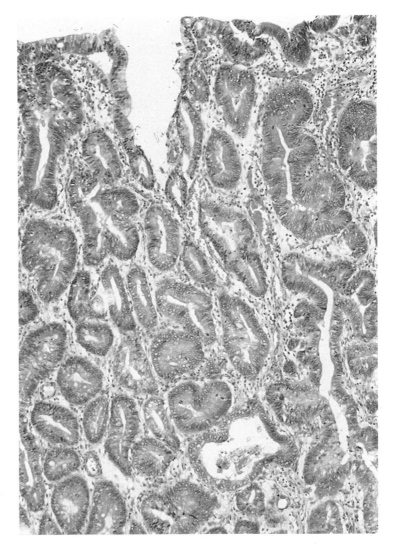

Moderate dysplasia in intestinal metaplasia, stomach

The tubules are closely apposed, as a result of branching and budding, but not yet back to back (see Fig. 43).

H&E. ×100.

Fig. 43
*Moderate dysplasia in
intestinal metaplasia,
stomach*

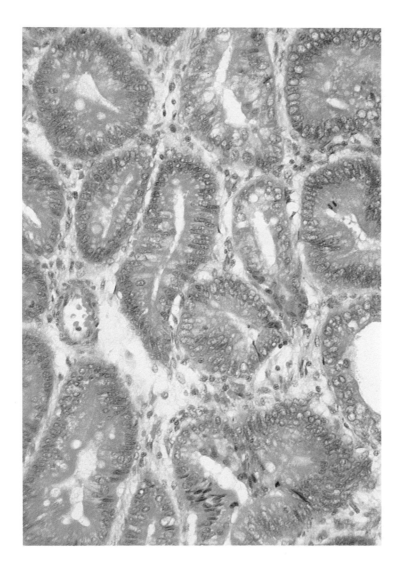

Moderate dysplasia in intestinal metaplasia, stomach

The nuclei are enlarged, ovoid and crowded. The chromatin is finely stippled, rather than coarsely clumped, and polarity is retained. The columnar cells show an eosinophilic cytoplasm and there are scattered goblet cells. The appearances are those of moderate dysplasia and may be compared with Fig. 25 which shows mild dysplasia within an intestinalized epithelium.

H&E. ×250.

Fig. 44
*Severe dysplasia in flat
gastric mucosa*

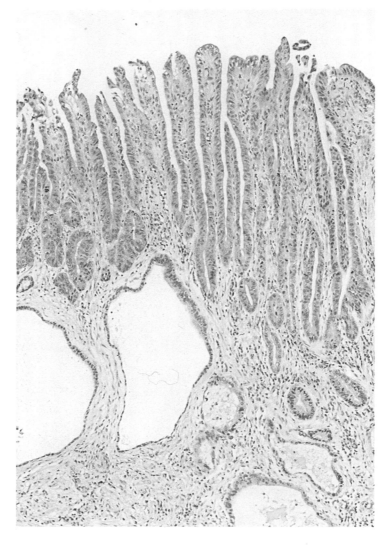

Severe dysplasia in flat gastric mucosa

The lesion arises within an atrophic mucosa. The crypts are straight
and closely aligned, but not yet back to back. Cystic change is
present (see Fig. 45).

H&E. ×100.

Fig. 45
*Severe dysplasia in flat
gastric mucosa*

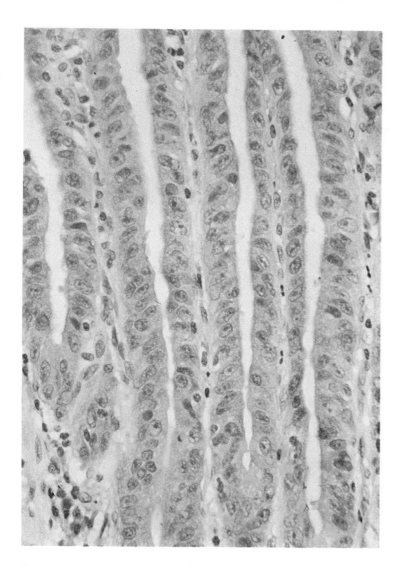

Severe dysplasia in flat gastric mucosa

The crypts are lined by low columnar cells with a pale eosinophilic
cytoplasm. The nuclei are enlarged, vesicular, and vary in size and
shape. Nuclear polarity is lost.

H&E. ×400.

Fig. 46
Severe dysplasia in flat gastric mucosa

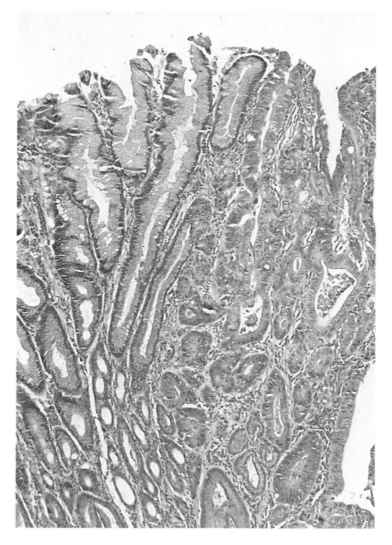

Severe dysplasia in flat gastric mucosa

Relatively normal gastric mucosa on the left contrasts with the architectural disorder on the right. The crypts show complex branching and back to back arrangements (see Fig. 47).

H&E. ×100.

Fig. 47
*Severe dysplasia in flat
gastric mucosa*

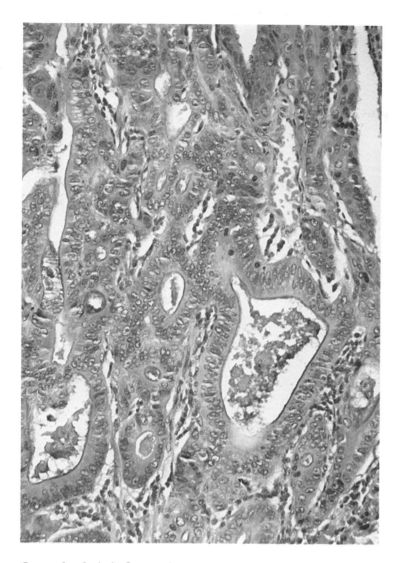

Severe dysplasia in flat gastric mucosa

The crypts are lined by eosinophilic columnar cells with a brush border. The nuclei are enlarged, vesicular and pleomorphic with focal loss of polarity. There are no goblet cells. Definite invasion of the lamina propria is not observed but the distinction from intra-mucosal carcinoma is not easily made. More obvious infiltrating carcinoma was present in other parts of the section.

H&E. ×250.

Fig. 48
*Moderate dysplasia
with villous
configuration, stomach*

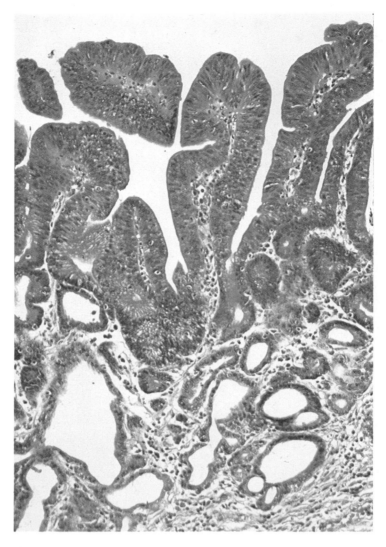

Moderate dysplasia with villous configuration, stomach

Villi are lined by tall, deeply basophilic cells. The underlying mucosa shows cystic atrophy (see Fig. 49).

H&E. ×160.

Fig. 49
*Moderate dysplasia
with villous
configuration, stomach*

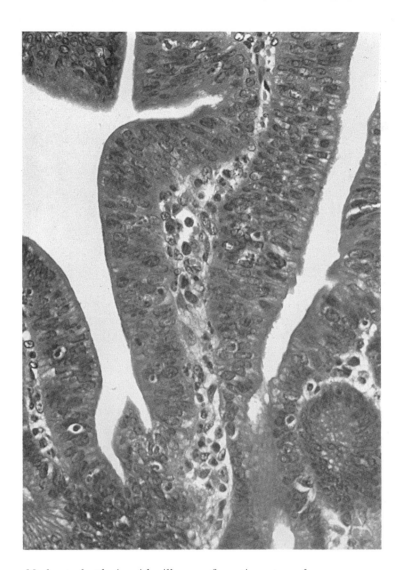

Moderate dysplasia with villous configuration, stomach

Nuclei are enlarged, hyperchromatic and pseudostratified.

H&E. ×400.

Fig. 50
*Severe dysplasia
amounting to
intramucosal
carcinoma, stomach*

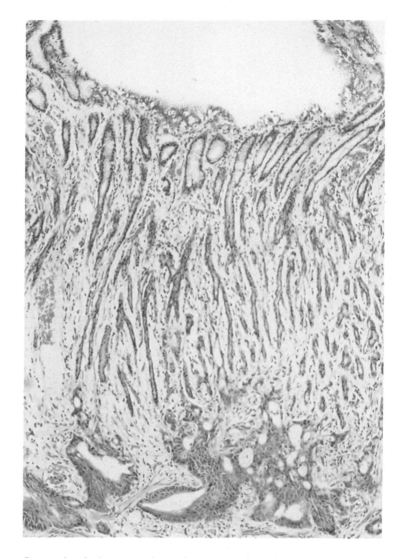

Severe dysplasia amounting to intramucosal carcinoma, stomach

The fundic glands are stretched into thin, branched ribbons within an oedematous lamina propria. More obvious carcinomatous elements occupy the lower third of the field (see Fig. 51).

H&E. ×100.

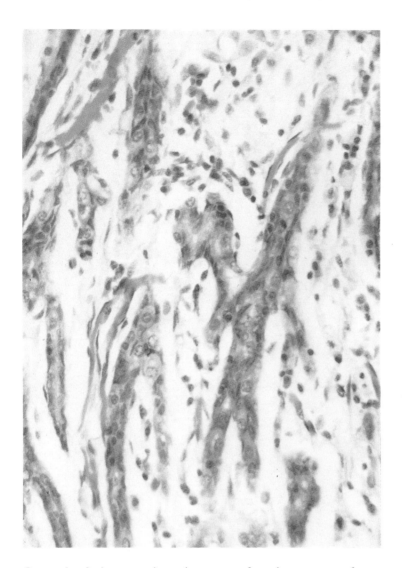

Severe dysplasia amounting to intramucosal carcinoma, stomach

It is possible to discern parietal cells within the branched, disorganized fundic glands. The cytology is bland, but the architectural changes indicate the correct diagnosis.

H&E. ×400.

Fig. 52
Tubular adenoma,
stomach

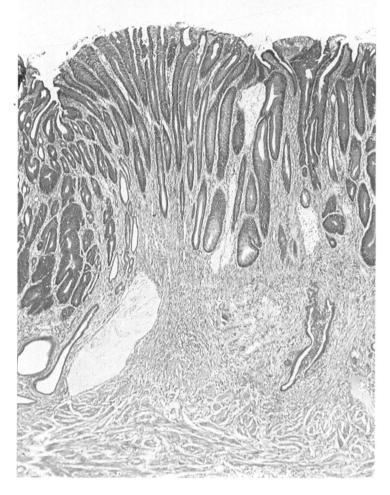

Tubular adenoma, stomach

The lesion, which presented as a sessile polyp, is composed of darkly staining tubules with relatively little branching. Cystic glands occupy the lower part of the field (see Fig. 53).

H&E. ×40.

Fig. 53
Tubular adenoma,
stomach

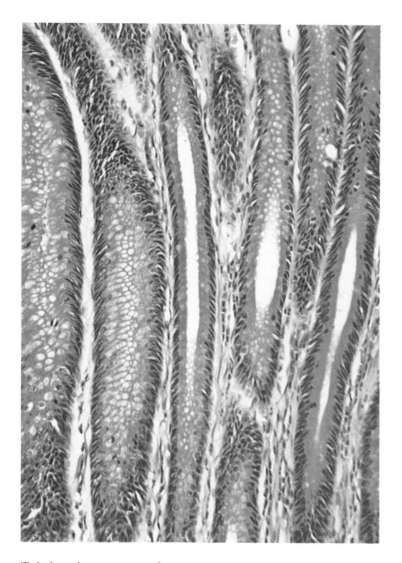

Tubular adenoma, stomach

The crowded tubules are lined by columnar cells secreting small amounts of mucus. The nuclei are elongated and crowded but regular in size and shape. Polarity is maintained. This represents mild dysplasia.

H&E. ×250.

Fig. 54

*Tubular adenoma—
junction with
non-neoplastic mucosa,
stomach*

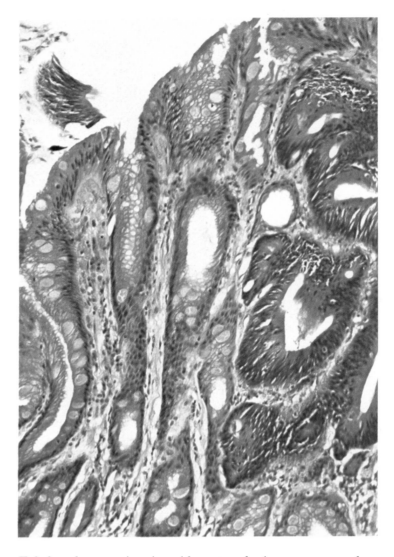

Tubular adenoma—junction with non-neoplastic mucosa, stomach

The non-neoplastic epithelium shows incomplete intestinal
metaplasia. The adenomatous epithelium reveals the occasional
vestigial goblet cell and deeply amphophilic columnar cells. The
nuclei are elongated and crowded, but not notably pleomorphic.
Polarity is retained and the changes amount to mild dysplasia.

H&E. ×160.

Fig. 55
*Tubulovillous
adenoma, stomach*

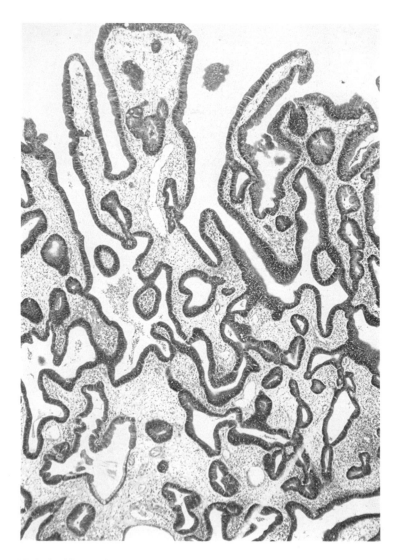

Tubulovillous adenoma, stomach

The villi and tubules are lined by darkly staining epithelium. The tubules show branching and budding, but are widely separated by an oedematous lamina propria (see Fig. 56).

H&E. ×40.

Fig. 56
*Tubulovillous
adenoma, stomach*

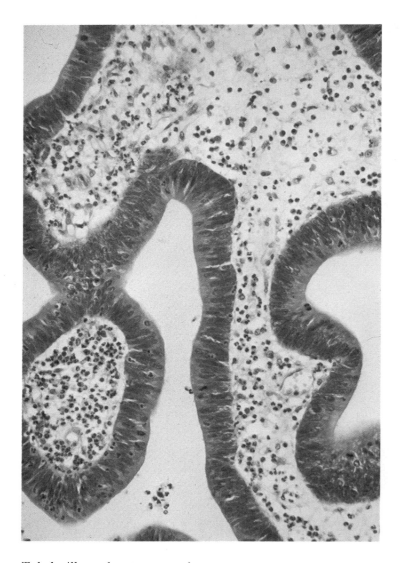

Tubulovillous adenoma, stomach

The nuclei are enlarged, ovoid and crowded with focal loss of polarity. The appearances amount to moderate dysplasia.

H&E. ×250.

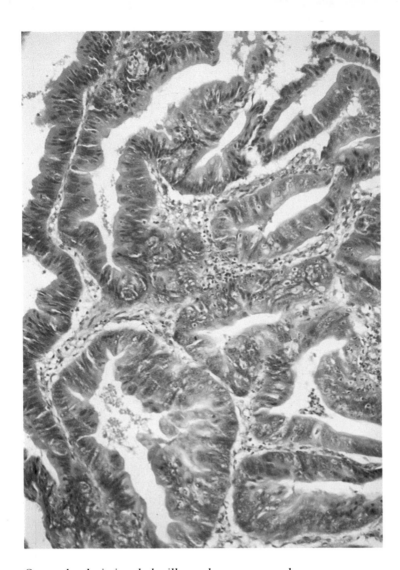

Fig. 57
*Severe dysplasia in
tubulovillous adenoma,
stomach*

Severe dysplasia in tubulovillous adenoma, stomach

This area occured as a small focus in the base of the
lesion shown in Figs. 55 and 56. The glands show an irregular,
papillary configuration and are arranged back to back. The nuclei
reveal pleomorphism and focal loss of polarity.

H&E. ×250.

Fig. 58

Tubulovillous adenoma—junction with gastric mucosa

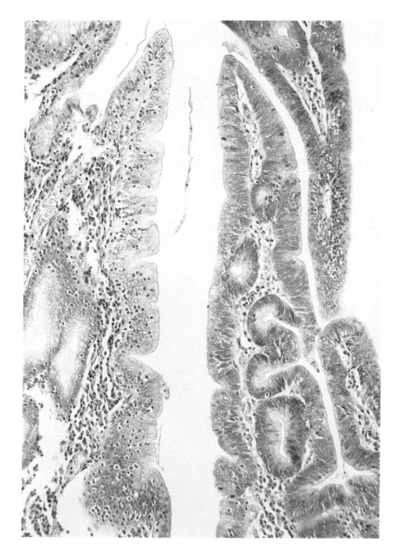

Tubulovillous adenoma—junction with gastric mucosa

The gastric mucosa on the left shows regenerative change due to active gastritis. The adenoma is lined by moderately dysplastic epithelium in which the nuclei are ovoid, enlarged hyperchromatic and crowded, but uniform in size and shape (see Fig. 59 and 60).

H&E. ×160.

Fig. 59
*Tubulovillous
adenoma—junction
with gastric mucosa
(mucins)*

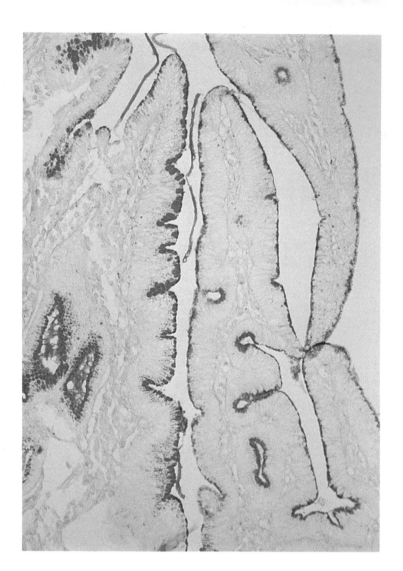

Tubulovillous adenoma—junction with gastric mucosa (mucins)

Gastric mucosa (left) secretes neutral mucins (red) and the
adenomatous epithelium (right) secretes acid mucins (blue).

Alcian blue/diastase PAS. ×160.

Fig. 60
*Tubulovillous
adenoma—junction
with gastric mucosa
(mucins)*

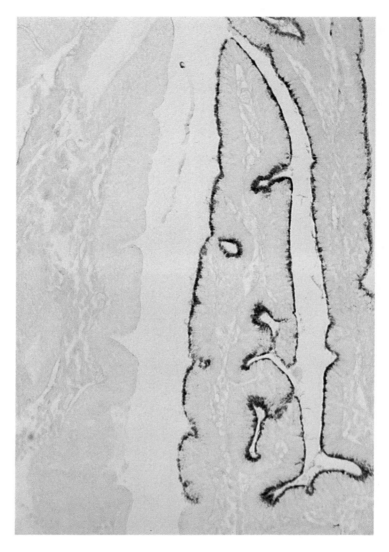

Tubulovillous adenoma—junction with gastric mucosa (mucins)

Neutral mucins (left) are unreactive whereas sulphomucins (right) give a brown reaction product.

High iron diamine/Alcian blue. ×160.

Fig. 61
Villous adenoma,
stomach

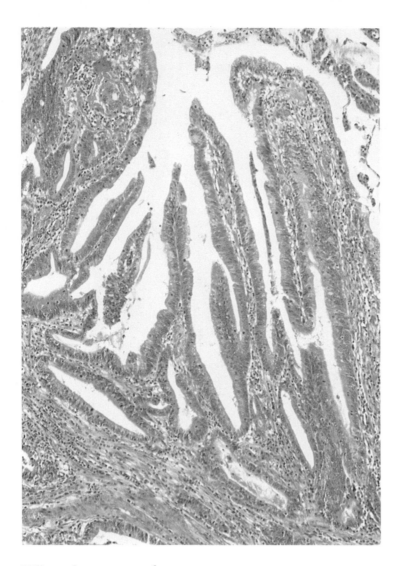

Villous adenoma, stomach

This represents part of a large papillary lesion which was associated with an underlying carcinoma (see Fig. 62).

H&E. ×120.

Fig. 62
Villous adenoma,
stomach

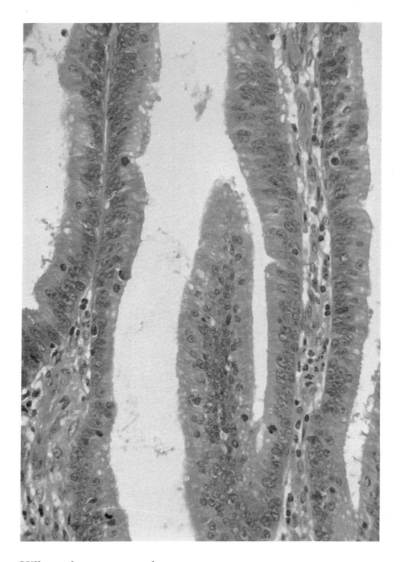

Villous adenoma, stomach

The villi are covered by amphophilic columnar cells which secrete small amounts of mucus. The nuclei are round and vesicular with a small nucleolus, but show neither pleomorphism nor loss of polarity. The appearances are those of mild cytological atypia.

H&E. ×400.

Fig. 63
*Hyperplastic polyp,
stomach*

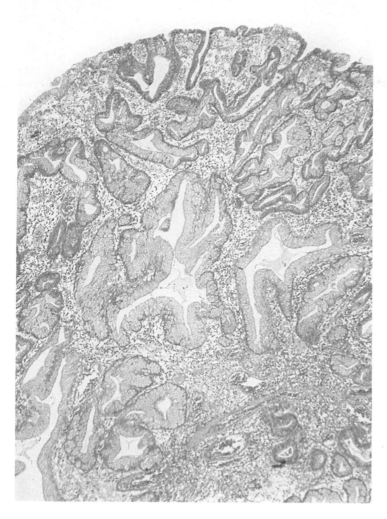

Hyperplastic polyp, stomach

The polyp includes gastric foveolar epithelium showing
architectural disorganization and the formation of complex
geographical outlines. The lamina propria is oedematous and
infiltrated with chronic inflammatory cells (see Fig. 64)

H&E. ×40.

Fig. 64
*Hyperplastic polyp,
stomach*

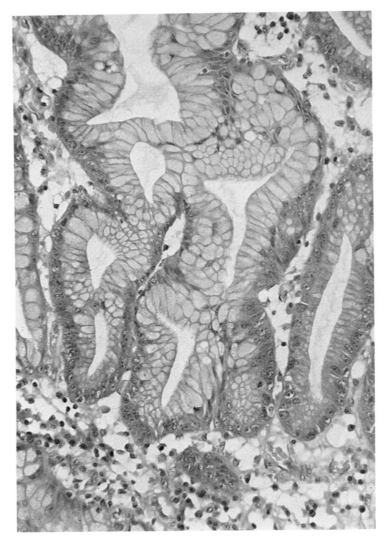

Hyperplastic polyp, stomach

The disorganized crypts are lined by essentially normal gastric foveolar epithelium.

H&E. ×250.

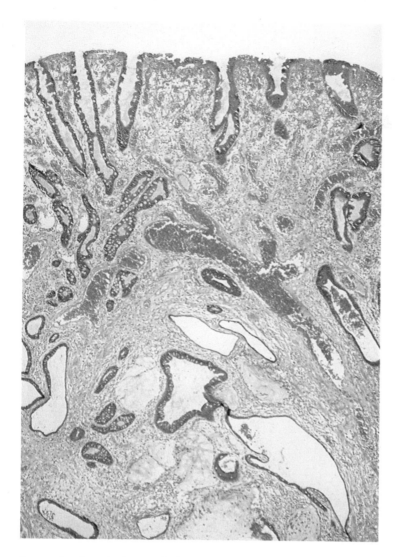

Incomplete intestinal metaplasia in hyperplastic polyp, stomach

This was one of the many large hyperplastic polyps. The crypts are set in an oedematous, congested lamina propria. Some show cystic change (see Fig. 66).

H&E. ×40.

Fig. 66

Incomplete intestinal metaplasia in hyperplastic polyp, stomach

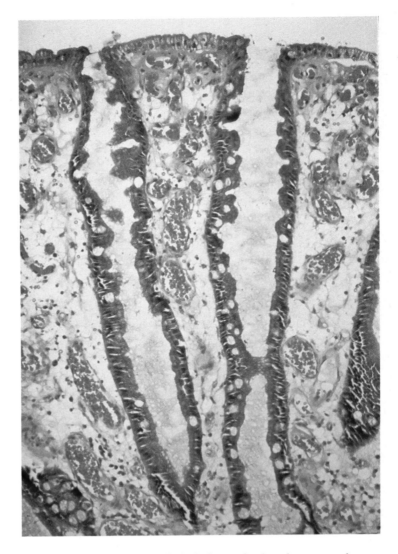

Incomplete intestinal metaplasia in hyperplastic polyp, stomach

The crypts are lined by deeply amphophilic columnar cells secreting very small amounts of mucus. Goblet cells are present. The appearances indicate regenerative change in intestinal metaplasia.

H&E. ×250.

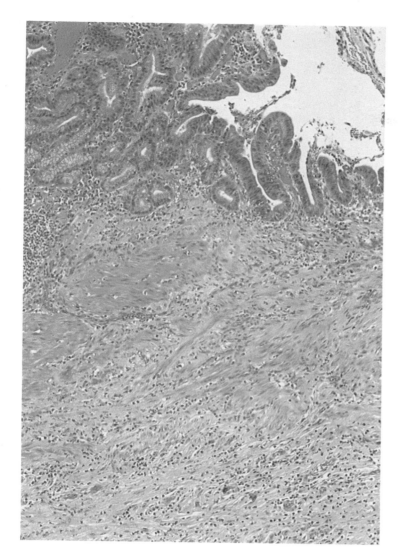

Regenerating epithelium relining benign peptic ulcer, stomach

A peptic ulcer which has destroyed the gastric wall is being relined by columnar epithelium showing dark, amphophilic cytoplasm (see Fig. 68).

H&E. ×100.

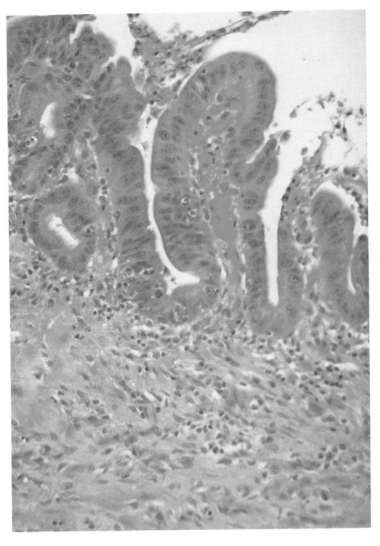

Regenerative epithelium relining benign peptic ulcer, stomach

The nuclei are enlarged and show focal loss of polarity. However, the clinical context and presence of active inflammation indicate the changes to be regenerative.

H&E. ×250.

Fig. 69
Ménétrier's disease,
stomach

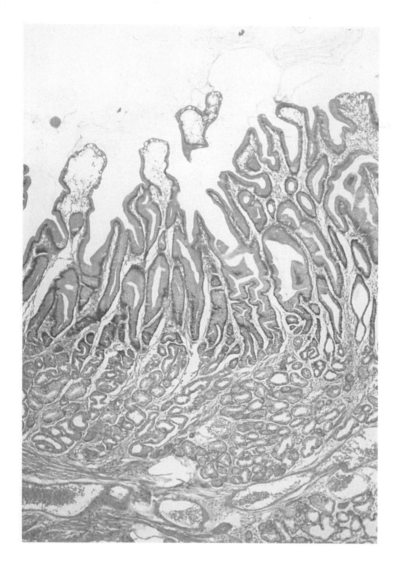

Ménétrier's disease, stomach

There is marked foveolar hyperplasia. This is accompanied by fundic gland atrophy and pyloric metaplasia.

H&E. ×40.

Fig. 70
*Ménétrier's disease,
stomach*

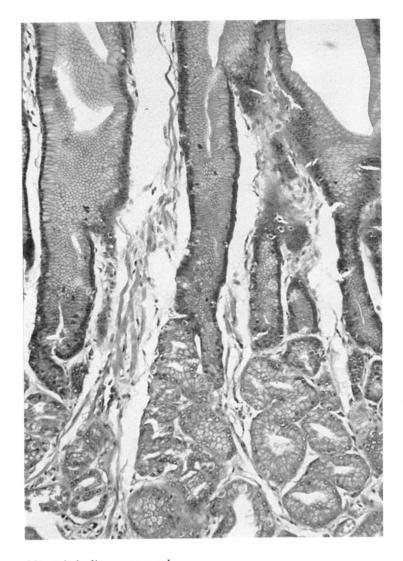

Ménétrier's disease, stomach

The lengthened foveolae are lined by a normal population of columnar mucous cells. Parietal cells are sparse and there is pyloric metaplasia. Strands of smooth muscle within the lamina propria are conspicuous. There is no dysplasia.

H&E. ×160.

Fig. 71
*Reactive change in
chronic active gastritis*

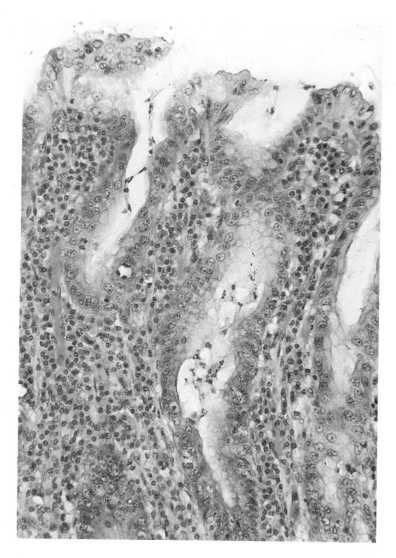

Reactive change in chronic active gastritis

The foveolar columnar cells show reduced mucus secretion and the
nuclei are enlarged and vesicular with a prominent nucleolus.
However, the nuclear membrane is delicate and there is neither
pleomorphism nor hyperchromatism. These reactive changes may
be mistaken for dysplasia.

H&E. ×250.

Fig. 72
*Regenerative change in
intestinal metaplasia,
stomach*

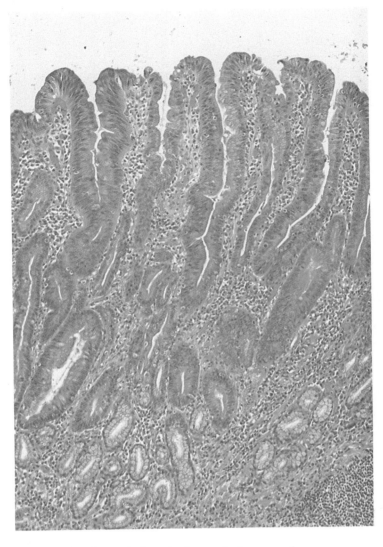

Regenerative change in intestinal metaplasia, stomach

There is active chronic gastritis with extensive intestinal metaplasia
(see Fig. 73).

H&E. ×100.

Fig. 73
*Regenerative change in
intestinal metaplasia,
stomach*

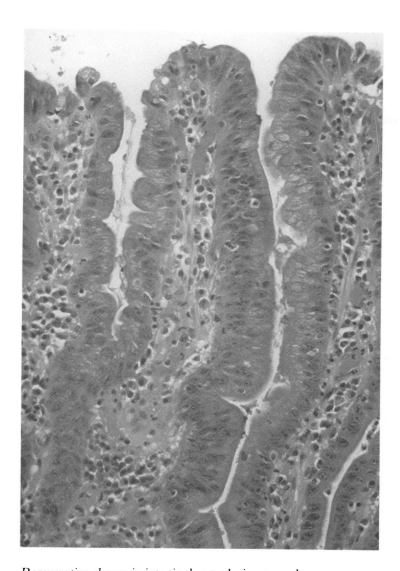

Regenerative change in intestinal metaplasia, stomach

The nuclei are enlarged, elongated and crowded and show focal loss
of polarity. The absence of architectural change and the presence
of active gastritis favour a diagnosis of regenerative change rather
than dysplasia.

H&E. ×250.

Fig. 74
*Fundic gland cysts,
stomach*

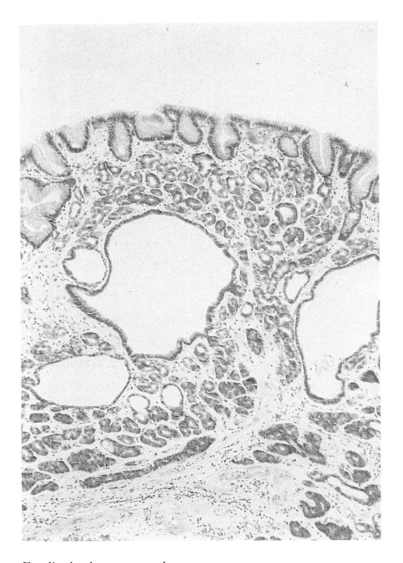

Fundic gland cysts, stomach

These lesions (which usually present as multiple small polyps in the body of the stomach) are not precancerous but may be associated with adenomatosis (familial polyposis coli). There is cystic dilatation of the fundic glands.

H&E. ×100.

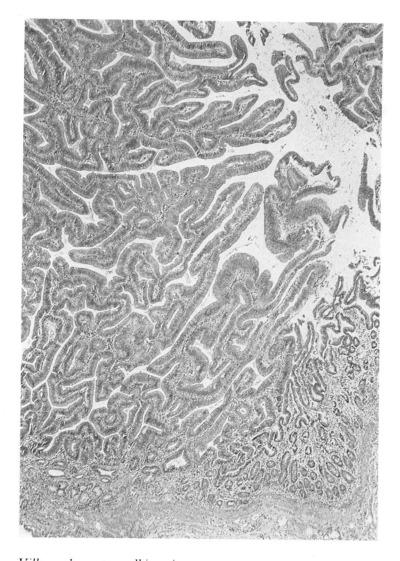

Fig. 75
*Villous adenoma, small
intestine*

Villous adenoma, small intestine

Normal small intestinal epithelium to the right adjoins a large
villous tumour (see Fig. 76).

H&E. ×40.

Fig. 76
*Villous adenoma, small
intestine*

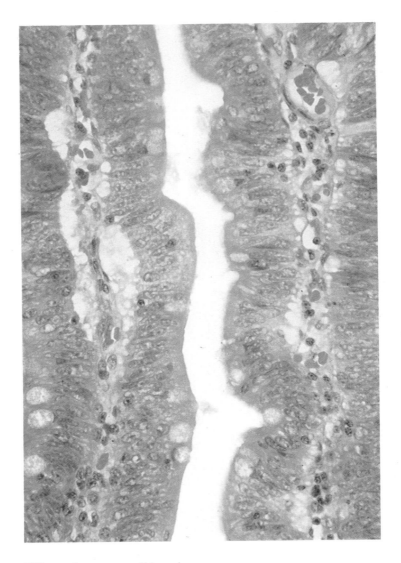

Villous adenoma, small intestine

The slender villi are lined by a mildly to moderately dysplastic epithelium comprising goblet cells and eosinophilic columnar cells. The nuclei are enlarged, elongated and vesicular, though they show little variation in size or shape.

H&E. ×250.

Fig. 77
*Villous adenoma in
adenomatosis, small
intestine*

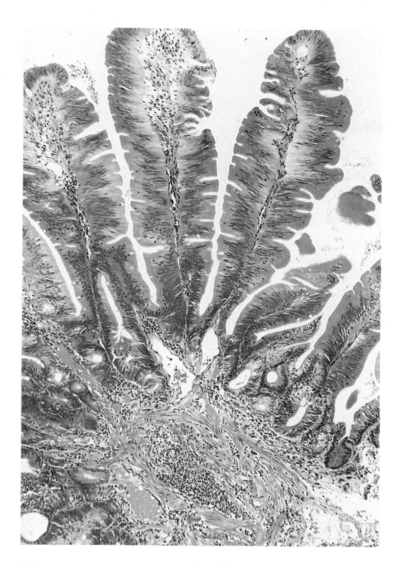

Villous adenoma in adenomatosis, small intestine

The villi are taller and broader than usual. They are lined by tall
columnar cells with an eosinophilic cytoplasm. Nuclei are crowded
and elongated, but small and lacking in pleomorphism. The
appearances are those of mild dysplasia.

H&E. ×100.

Fig. 78
*Peutz–Jeghers polyp,
small intestine*

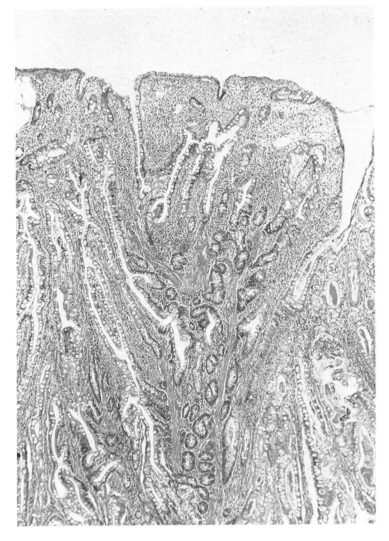

Peutz–Jeghers polyp, small intestine

The polyp shows a complex, papillary configuration, with strands of smooth muscle passing into the lamina propria.

H&E. ×40.

Fig. 79
*Peutz–Jeghers polyp,
small intestine*

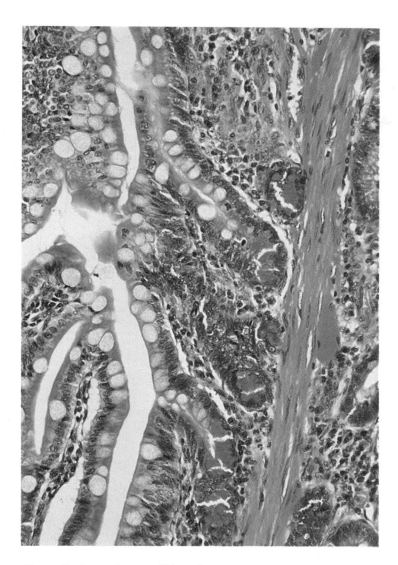

Peutz–Jeghers polyp, small intestine

The epithelial lining includes mature absorptive cells, goblet cells and Paneth cells. There is no dysplasia.

H&E. ×160.

Fig. 80
*Dysplasia in Crohn's
disease, small intestine*

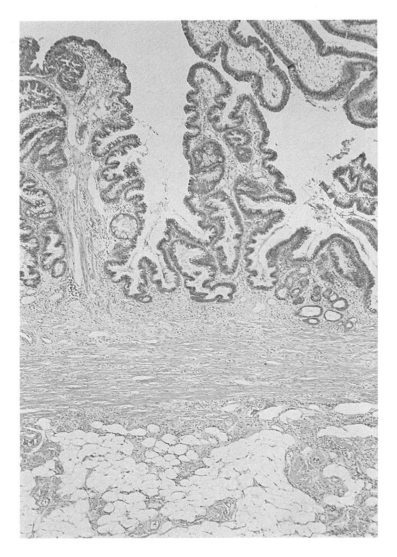

Dysplasia in Crohn's disease, small intestine

The muscularis mucosae is thickened and the submucosa shows fibrosis, fatty infiltration and mild chronic inflammation. (More characteristic features of Crohn's disease were identified in other parts of the specimen.) The epithelium covers frond-like, papillary processes (see Fig. 81).

H&E. ×40.

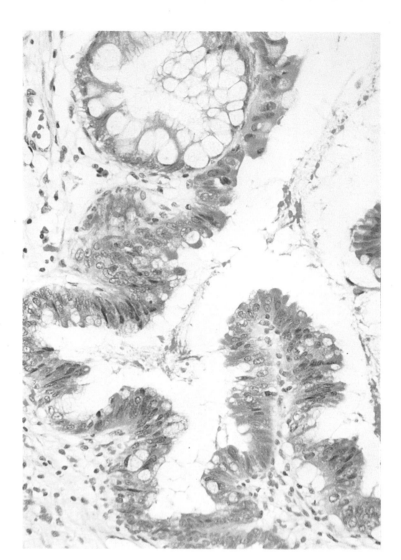

Fig. 81
*Dysplasia in Crohn's
disease, small intestine*

Dysplasia in Crohn's disease, small intestine

The epithelial lining includes columnar cells and goblet cells. The nuclei are enlarged and crowded and show focal loss of polarity. The appearances amount to mild dysplasia.

H&E. ×250.

Fig. 82
*Tubular adenoma,
appendix*

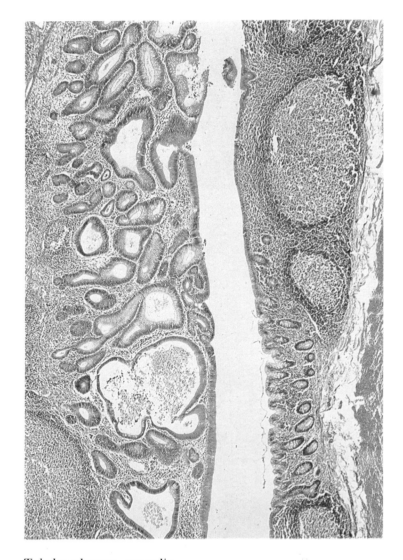

Tubular adenoma, appendix

This presented in a case of adenomatosis (familial polyposi coli). In the left half of the field, the mucosa is thickened and includes branched, dilated tubules (see Fig. 83).

H&E. ×40.

Fig. 83
Tubular adenoma,
appendix

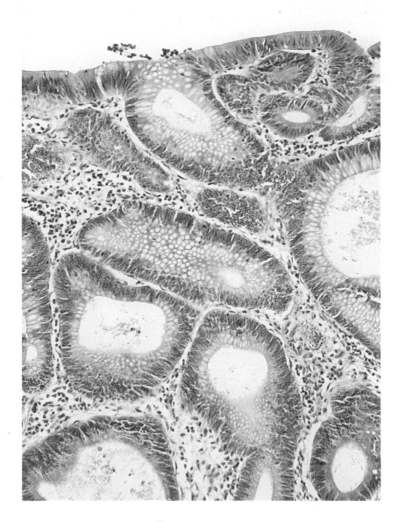

Tubular adenoma, appendix

There is a slight reduction in mucus within the goblet cells and the nuclei are increased in size and crowded. Polarity is well maintained and the changes amount to mild dysplasia.

H&E. ×160.

Fig. 84
Cystadenoma, appendix

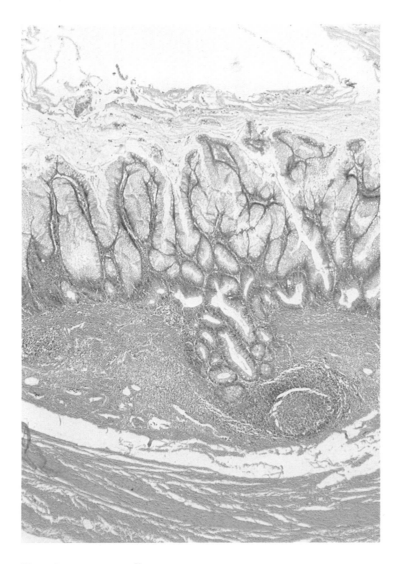

Cystadenoma, appendix

This appendix was dilated and filled with mucus. The mucosa is thickened and comprises branched tubules lined by tall mucous cells. There is pseudoinvasion (see Fig. 85).

H&E. ×40.

Fig. 85
Cystadenoma, appendix

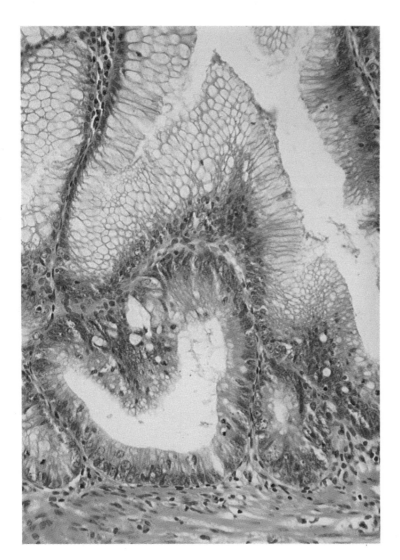

Cystadenoma, appendix

Dysplasia is very mild and confined to the crypt base region.

H&E. ×250.

Fig. 86
Cystadenoma (villous), appendix

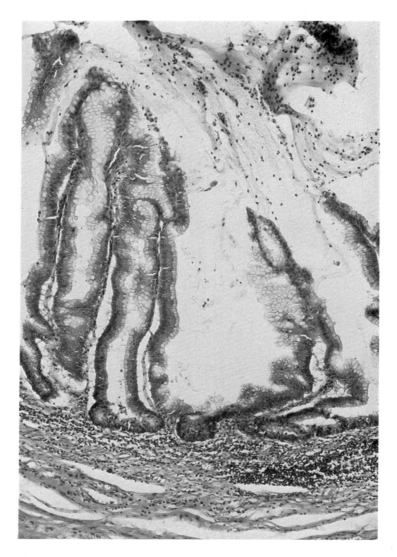

Cystadenoma (villous), appendix

Slender villi lined by mucus-secreting cells project into the lumen of the appendix. Dysplasia is mild, but there was an associated mucinous adenocarcinoma (not shown).

H&E. ×100.

Fig. 87
Hyperplastic polyp,
appendix

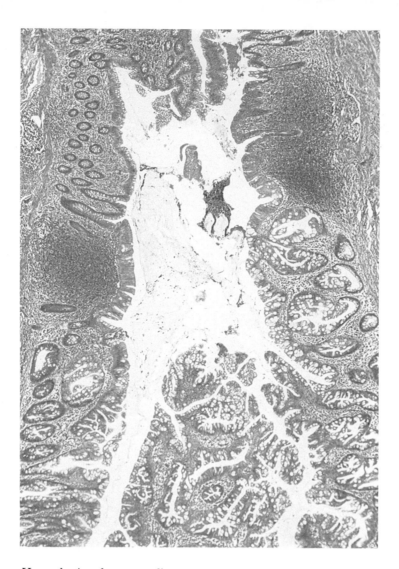

Hyperplastic polyp, appendix

The hyperplastic polyp lining the tip of this appendix shows an exaggerated papillary configuration and could be mistaken for a villous adenoma (see Fig. 88).

H&E. ×40.

Fig. 88
Hyperplastic polyp,
appendix

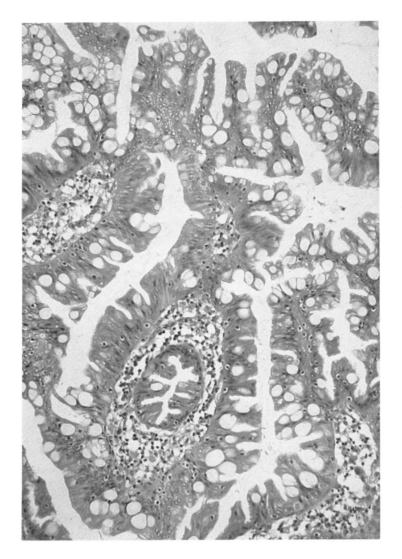

Hyperplastic polyp, appendix

A typical serrated configuration and lack of cytological atypia are shown.

H&E. ×160.

Fig. 89
Tubular adenoma,
colorectum

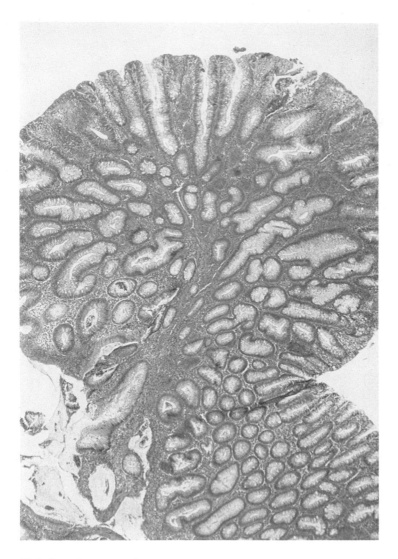

Tubular adenoma, colorectum

The tubules show branching and budding and appear relatively crowded (see Fig. 90).

H&E. ×40.

Fig. 90
Tubular adenoma,
colorectum

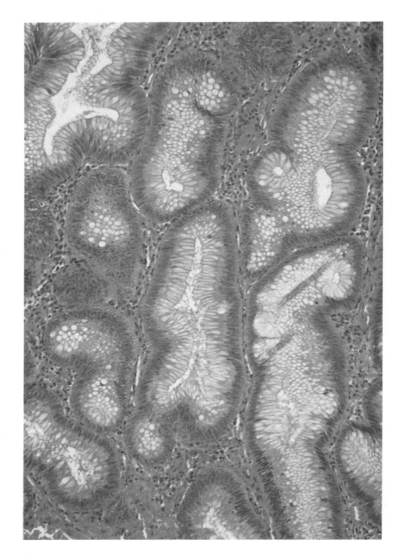

Tubular adenoma, colorectum

The nuclei are slightly enlarged, ovoid and a little crowded, but polarity is retained. The goblet cells are tall, crowded and probably show a slight reduction in mucus content in relation to their size.

H&E. ×160.

Fig. 91
Tubular adenoma,
colorectum

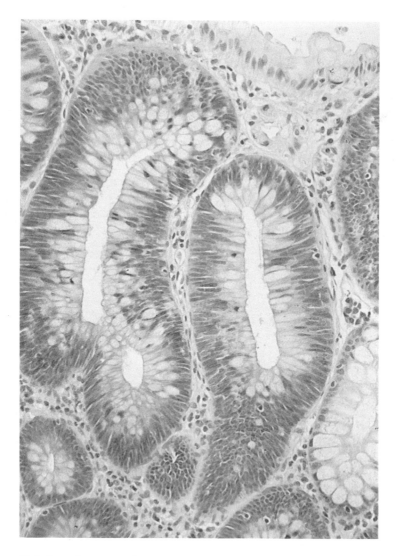

Tubular adenoma, colorectum

The nuclei show focal loss of polarity and there is slight depletion of mucus. Dysplasia is more marked than in Fig. 90, but still mild.

H&E. ×250.

Fig. 92
Flat tubular adenoma,
colorectum

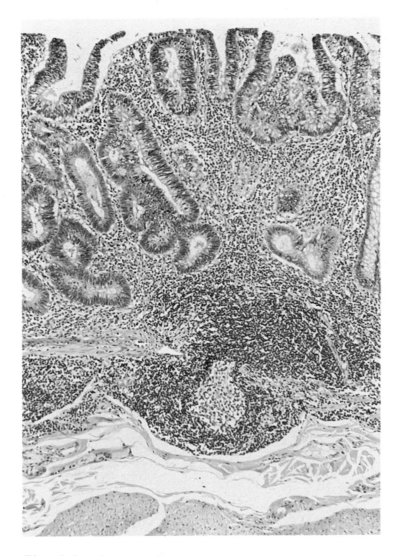

Flat tubular adenoma, colorectum

Entirely flat adenomas are unusual but serve to emphasize that epithelial dysplasia (rather than the elevation of a lesion) is the principal indicator of neoplastic change (see Fig. 93).

H&E. ×100.

Fig. 93
*Flat tubular adenoma,
colorectum*

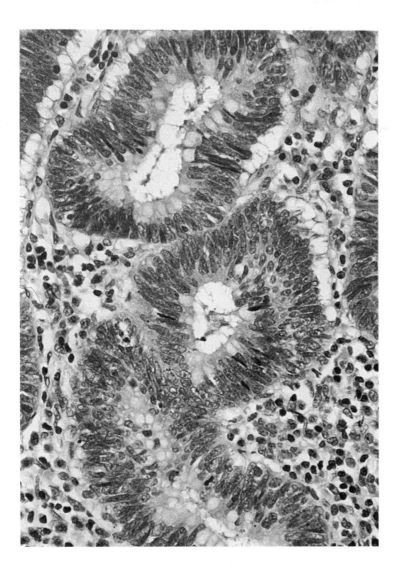

Flat tubular adenoma, colorectum

The neoplastic tubules are lined by an epithelium whose nuclei are elongated, hyperchromatic and pseudostratified. Polarity is still retained. The changes are those of moderate dysplasia.

H&E. ×250.

Fig. 94
Villous adenoma,
colorectum

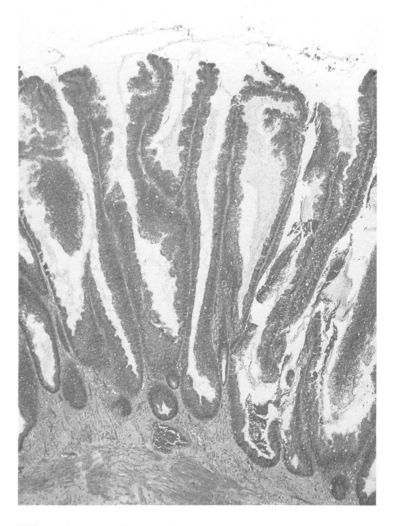

Villous adenoma, colorectum

Part of a large villous adenoma is shown. The intervillous columnar cells are not forming tubules and sit immediately above the muscularis mucosae (see Fig. 95).

H&E. ×40.

Fig. 95
Villous adenoma,
colorectum

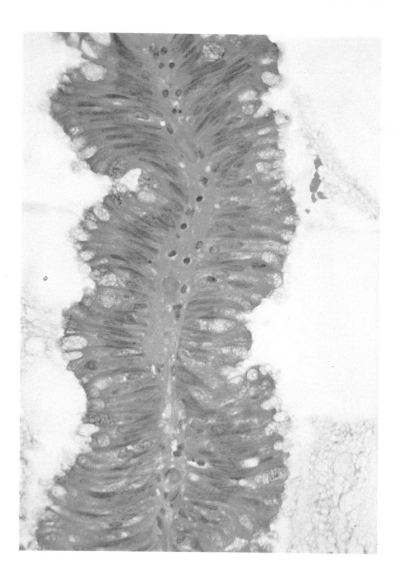

Villous adenoma, colorectum

The slender villi are covered by tall columnar cells, many of which contain small amounts of mucus. The nuclei are crowded and elongated but not pleomorphic. The cytological appearances are those of mild dysplasia.

H&E. ×400.

Fig. 96
Flat villous adenoma,
colorectum

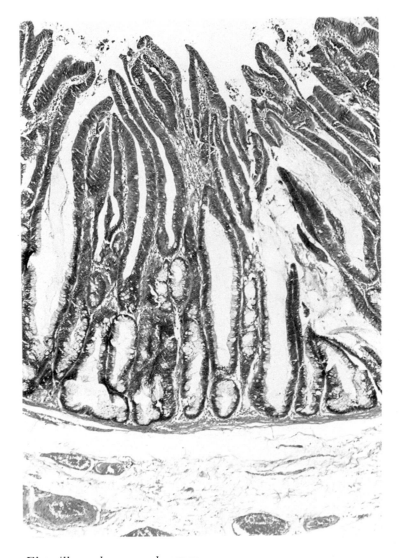

Flat villous adenoma, colorectum

This lesion appeared macroscopically as a slightly thickened, velvety mucosa bordering a colorectal carcinoma. It may be regarded as the villous counterpart of Fig. 92.

H&E. ×60.

Fig. 97
*Tubulovillous
adenoma, colorectum*

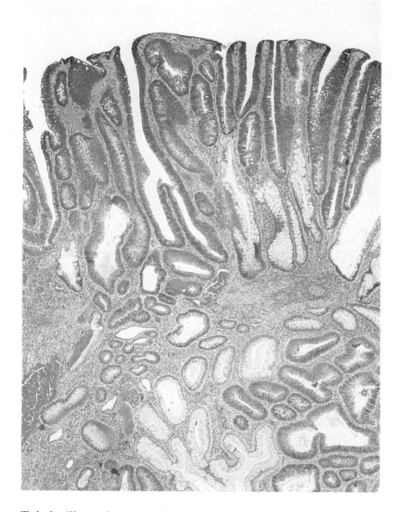

Tubulovillous adenoma, colorectum

The upper part of the lesion shows a predominantly villous
configuration, whereas branched tubules occupy the lower field
(see Fig. 98).

H&E. ×40.

Fig. 98
*Tubulovillous
adenoma, colorectum*

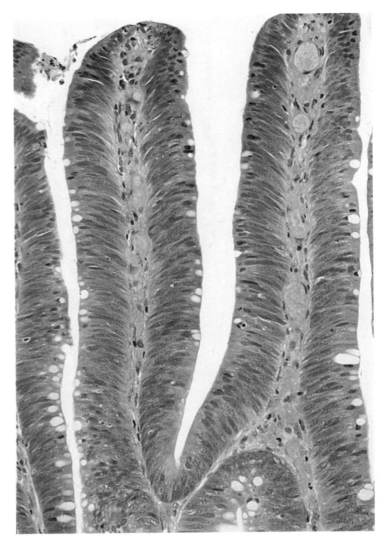

Tubulovillous adenoma, colorectum

The villi are covered by dark amphophilic columnar cells and immature goblet cells. The nuclei are elongated, hyperchromatic and pseudostratified with focal loss of polarity. These changes amount to moderate dysplasia.

H&E. ×250.

Fig. 99
*Dysplasia in flat
mucosa, colorectum*

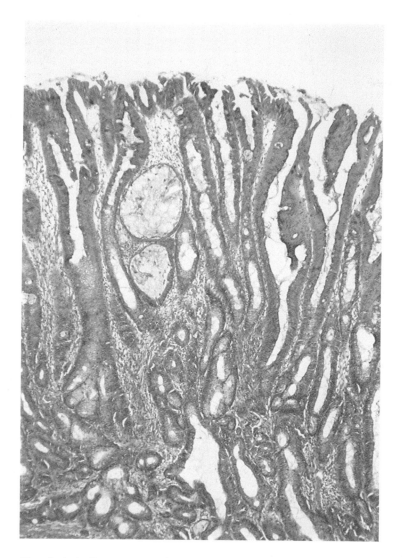

Dysplasia in flat mucosa, colorectum

The crypts are lengthened and show papillary infolding.
Branching and budding from the crypt base region has occurred
(see Fig. 100).

H&E. ×60.

Fig. 100
*Dysplasia in flat
mucosa, colorectum*

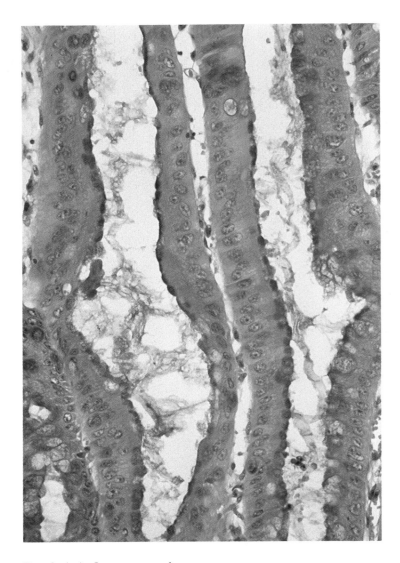

Dysplasia in flat mucosa, colorectum

The crypts are lined by eosinophilic columnar cells which secrete small amounts of acid mucus (basophilic with Ehrlich's haematoxylin). There are occasional goblet cells. The nuclei are round to oval and vesicular with a prominent nucleolus. This unusual form of dysplasia occurred in the immediate vicinity of a poorly differentiated mucinous carcinoma. The appearances are reminiscent of incomplete maturation (basal cell hyperplasia) in ulcerative colitis (compare with Fig. 128). Precise criteria for grading such forms of dysplasia have not been laid down.

H&E. ×250.

Fig. 101
Adenomatosis,
colorectum

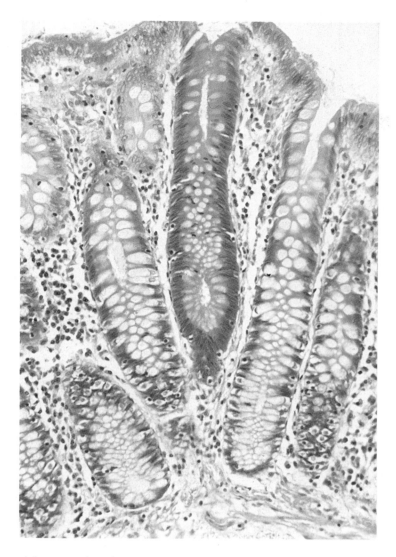

Adenomatosis, colorectum

Focal mild dysplasia involving a single crypt may be observed when apparently normal, non-polypoid mucosa is sampled from patients with adenomatosis (familial polyposis coli).

H&E. ×250.

Fig. 102
Adenomatosis,
colorectum

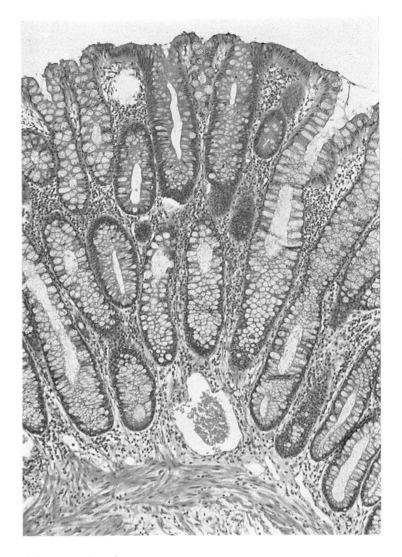

Adenomatosis, colorectum

Four adjacent crypts reveal very mild dysplasia, resulting in the formation of a microadenoma.

H&E. ×100.

Fig. 103
Adenomatosis,
colorectum

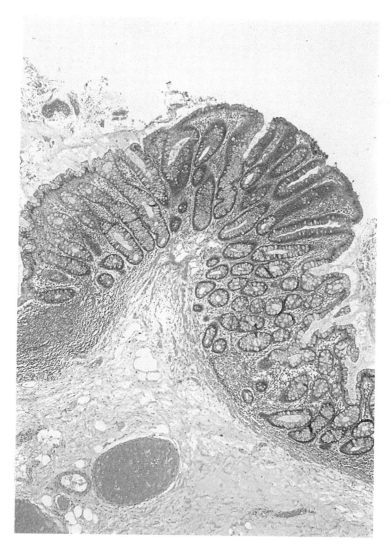

Adenomatosis, colorectum

Microadenomas of this size will form a small excrescence, visible to the naked eye.

H&E. ×100.

Fig. 104
Juvenile polyp,
colorectum

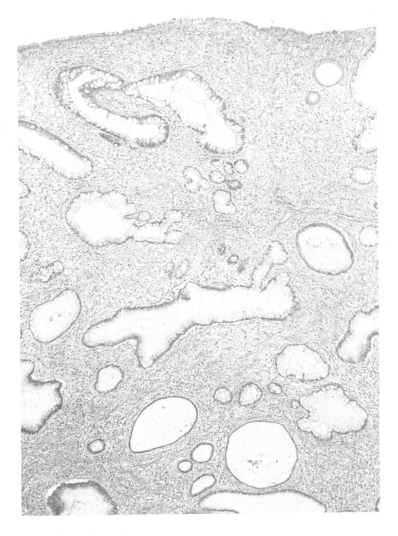

Juvenile polyp, colorectum

Crypts showing branching, budding and cystic change are embedded in a haphazard fashion in an oedematous lamina propria. The crypts are lined by normal colorectal epithelium.

H&E. ×40

Fig. 105
*Reactive change in
juvenile polyp, colorectum*

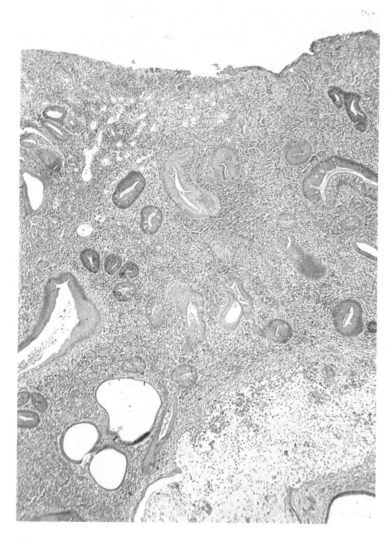

Reactive change in juvenile polyp, colorectum

Tubules are widely separated by a cellular, highly vascularized
stroma. A cystic crypt has ruptured, releasing its mucous contents
into the lamina propria (see Fig. 106).

H&E. ×40.

Fig. 106
*Reactive change in
juvenile polyp,
colorectum*

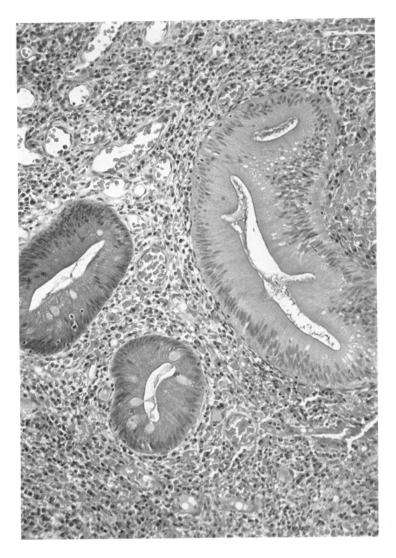

Reactive change in juvenile polyp, colorectum

The tubules are lined by columnar cells secreting tiny amounts of apical mucin (basophilic with Ehrlich's haematoxylin) and small numbers of goblet cells. The nuclei are elongated and crowded but remain small and uniform in size and shape. This mild failure in maturation is commonly observed in juvenile polyps and is likely to represent a form of reactive change. It is not known whether such foci are more prone to become dysplastic.

H&E. × 160.

Fig. 107
*Dysplasia in juvenile
polyp, colorectum*

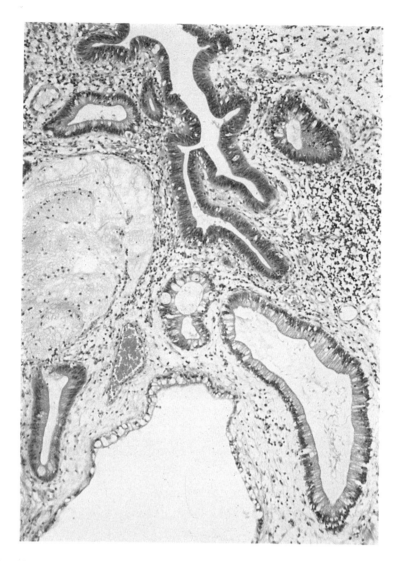

Dysplasia in juvenile polyp, colorectum

Some of the cystically dilated crypts are lined by normal colorectal
epithelium. Elsewhere, changes ranging from incomplete
maturation through to frank dysplasia are evident.

H&E. ×100.

Fig. 108
*Dysplasia in
juvenile polyp,
colorectum*

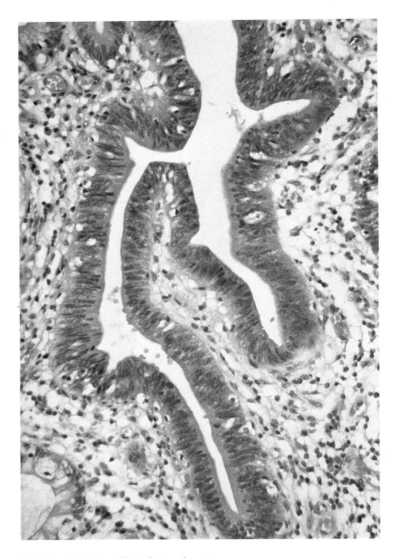

Dysplasia in juvenile polyp, colorectum

The nuclei are enlarged, hyperchromatic and pseudostratified.
The changes amount to moderate dysplasia.

H&E. ×100.

Fig. 109
*Dysplasia in juvenile
polyposis, colorectum*

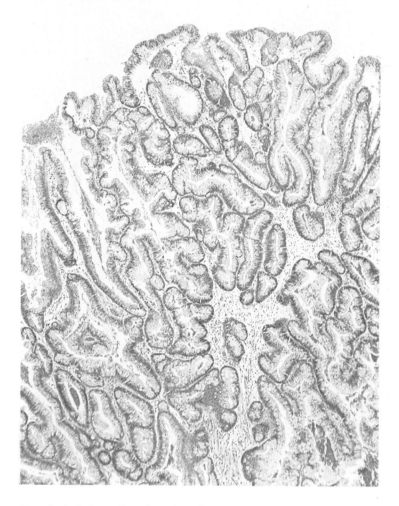

Dysplasia in juvenile polyposis, colorectum

This was one of the many polyps from a child followed up for
several years. In such relatively long-standing cases of juvenile
polyposis, the crypts may show complex budding and papillary
infoldings with a reduction in the amount of intervening lamina
propria (see Fig. 110).

H&E. ×40.

Fig. 110
*Dysplasia in juvenile
polyposis, colorectum*

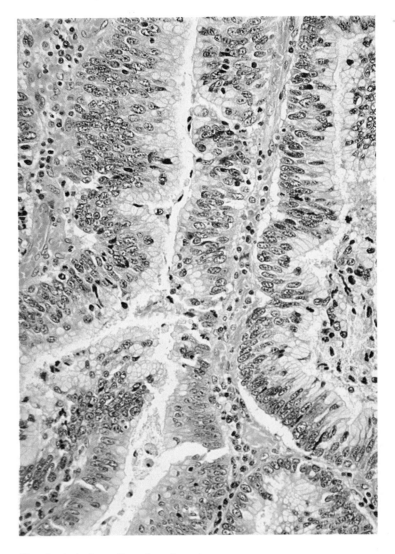

Dysplasia in juvenile polyposis, colorectum

This field was observed in a different part of the polyp illustrated in
Fig. 109. Nuclei are enlarged, hyperchromatic and show
pseudostratification, though polarity is retained. The cells secrete
small amounts of mucus.

H&E. ×250.

Fig. 111
*Pseudoinvasion in
hyperplastic polyp,
colorectum*

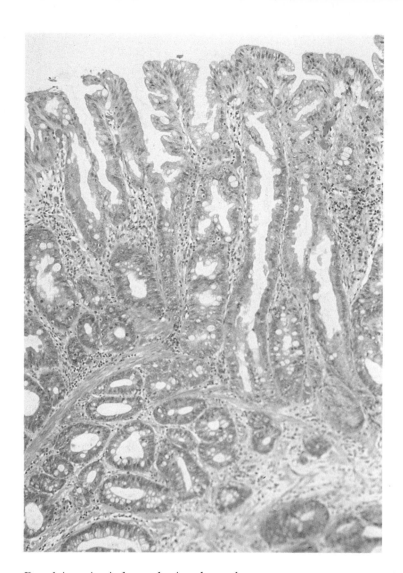

Pseudoinvasion in hyperplastic polyp, colorectum

The crypts show a serrated contour and are lined by small numbers
of goblet cells and columnar cells with pale, eosinophilic
cytoplasm. The muscularis mucosae appears frayed and
proliferated tubules are intermingled with fragments of smooth
muscle (see Fig. 112).

H&E. ×100.

Fig. 112
*Pseudoinvasion in
hyperplastic polyp,
colorectum*

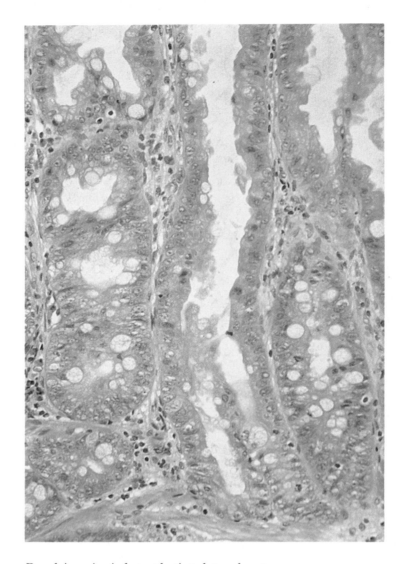

Pseudoinvasion in hyperplastic polyp, colorectum

The crypt base cells show round, vesicular nuclei and a prominent
nucleolus. At higher levels within the crypt, the nuclei are still
vesicular, but relatively small and with a delicate nuclear
membrane. Normal polarity is retained. These appearances do not
amount to dysplasia.

H&E. ×250.

Fig. 113
*Mild dysplasia in
hyperplastic polyp,
colorectum*

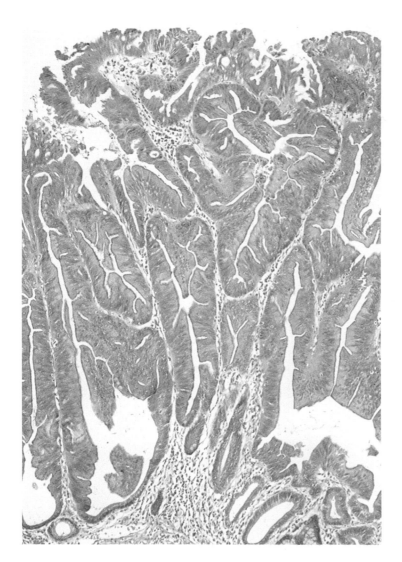

Mild dysplasia in hyperplastic polyp, colorectum

The lesion shows the configuration of a hyperplastic polyp, including the serrated outline and dilated crypt base region. Goblet cells are few in number. Dark, eosinophilic cells secreting small amounts of acid mucus (basophilic with Ehrlich's haematoxylin) predominate. The nuclei are elongated and crowded with slight pseudostratification.

H&E. ×100.

Fig. 114
*Chronic quiescent
ulcerative colitis*

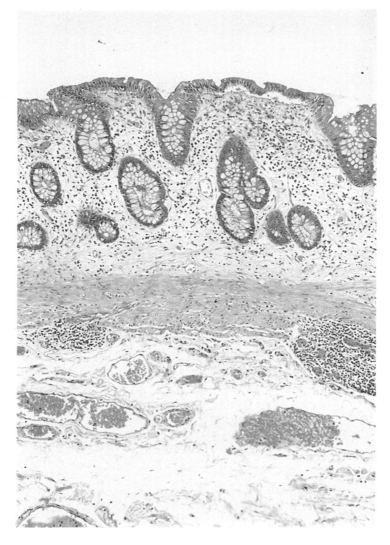

Chronic quiescent ulcerative colitis

The mucosa is atrophic and the crypts show mild architectural
changes, including shortfall. The muscularis mucosae is
thickened. These changes characterize long-standing ulcerative
colitis in remission. Dysplasia is not present.

H&E. ×100.

Fig. 115
Regenerative change in
active, follicular
ulcerative colitis

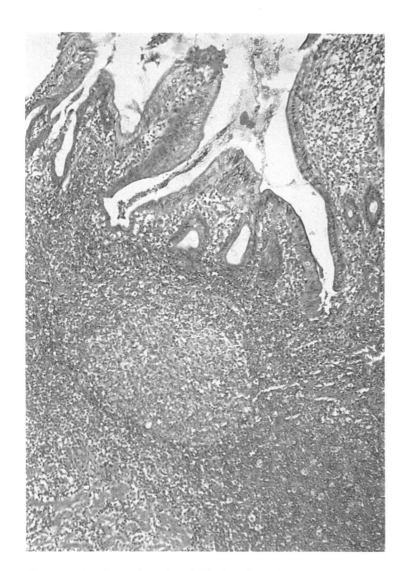

Regenerative change in active, follicular ulcerative colitis

There is marked regenerative distortion of the mucosa and a heavy lymphocytic infiltration within the lamina propria. A lymphoid follicle with a germinal centre is included. The surface epithelium shows goblet cell depletion.

H&E. ×100.

Fig. 116
*Regenerative change in
active ulcerative colitis*

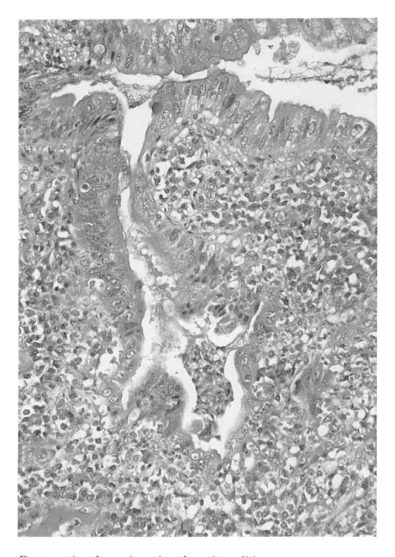

Regenerative change in active ulcerative colitis

The crypt epithelium reveals mucus depletion, and the nuclei are enlarged and vesicular and vary in size and shape. There is focal ulceration of the crypt lining and an early crypt abscess. In the presence of active, acute inflammation, the epithelial changes must be regarded as reactive.

H&E. ×250.

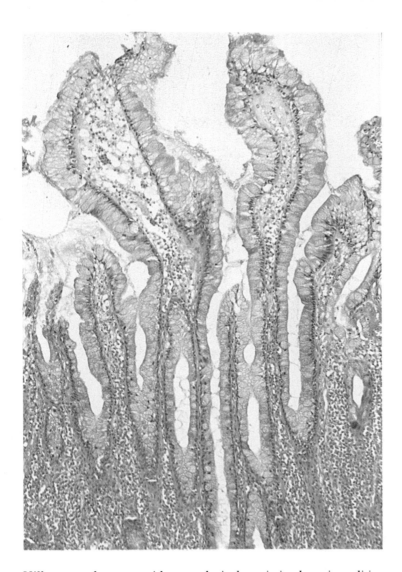

Fig. 117
*Villous growth pattern
with no cytological
atypia in ulcerative
colitis*

Villous growth pattern with no cytological atypia in ulcerative colitis

The villous processes are covered by tall mucous cells showing no cytological atypia. The clinical significance of this growth pattern has not been determined and such a lesion could be placed in the category 'indefinite' for dysplasia until its natural history is understood. Sometimes dysplasia is confined to the crypt region of such lesions, when the appearances recall Figs. 125 and 126.

H&E. ×100.

Fig. 118
*Mild villous dysplasia,
ulcerative colitis*

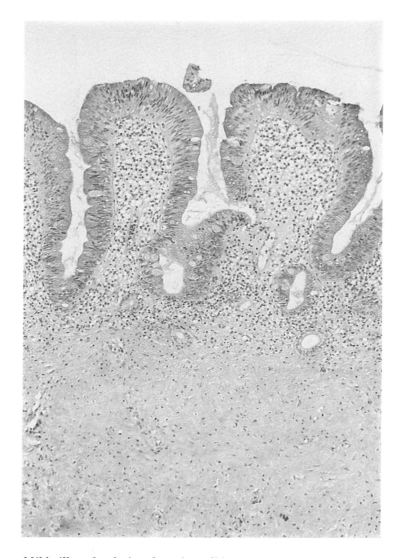

Mild villous dysplasia, ulcerative colitis

The villi illustrated are short and broad, but may also be tall and slender. In the latter instance, the appearances will be similar to the flat villous adenoma of the appendix (Fig. 86) or colorectum (Fig. 96). Detail of the lining epithelium is shown in Fig. 119.

H&E. ×100.

Fig. 119
*Mild villous dysplasia,
ulcerative colitis*

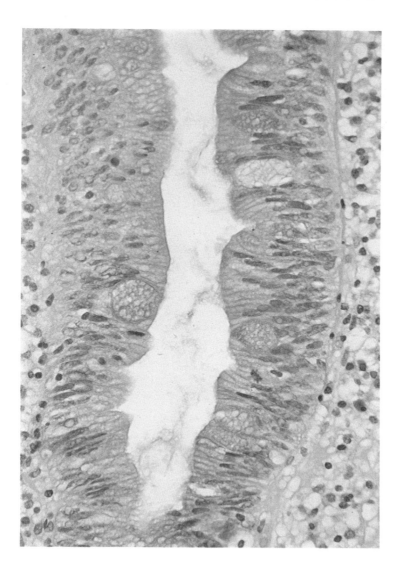

Mild villous dysplasia, ulcerative colitis

The villi are covered by tall columnar cells with a pale, eosinophilic cytoplasm and goblet cells. Nuclei are elongated and crowded, but with only focal loss of polarity.

H&E. ×400.

Fig. 120
*Moderate villous
dysplasia, ulcerative
colitis*

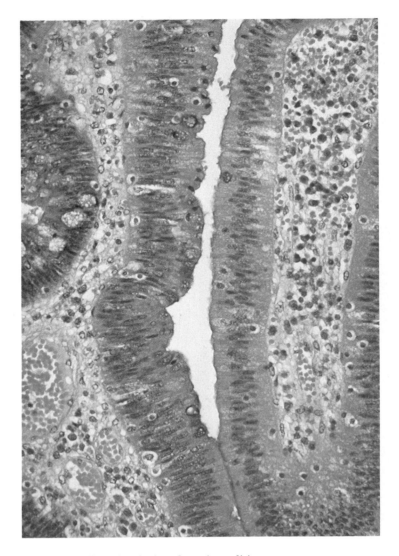

Moderate villous dysplasia, ulcerative colitis

The villi are covered by tall, amphophilic columnar cells and the occasional goblet cell. Nuclei are elongated, hyperchromatic and pseudostratified. The changes approach moderate dysplasia, but would be regarded as low grade in the two grade system.

H&E. ×250.

Fig. 121
*Severe villous
dysplasia, ulcerative
colitis*

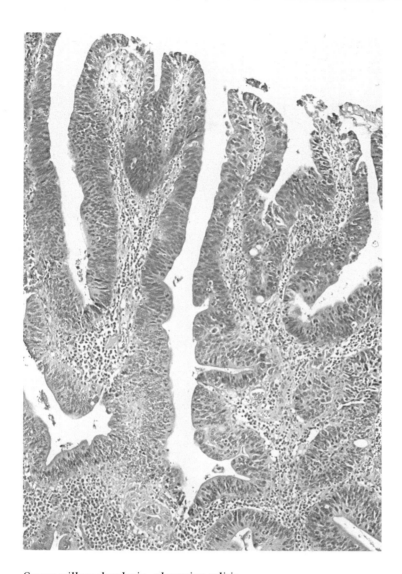

Severe villous dysplasia, ulcerative colitis

Tubules bud into the lips of the villi, producing club-shaped
structures (see Fig. 122).

H&E. ×100.

Fig. 122
*Severe villous
dysplasia, ulcerative
colitis*

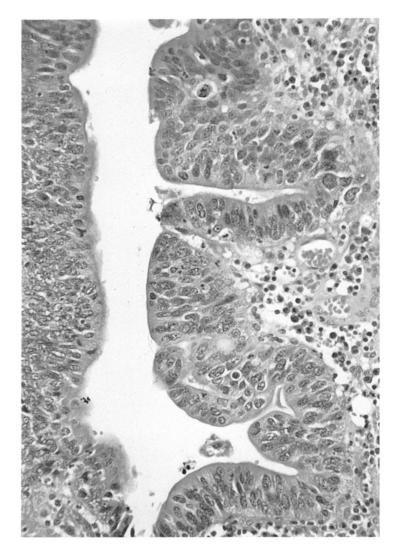

Severe villous dysplasia, ulcerative colitis

The nuclei are enlarged, pleomorphic and hyperchromatic and show loss of polarity.

H&E. ×250.

Fig. 123
Mild dysplasia in flat mucosa, ulcerative colitis

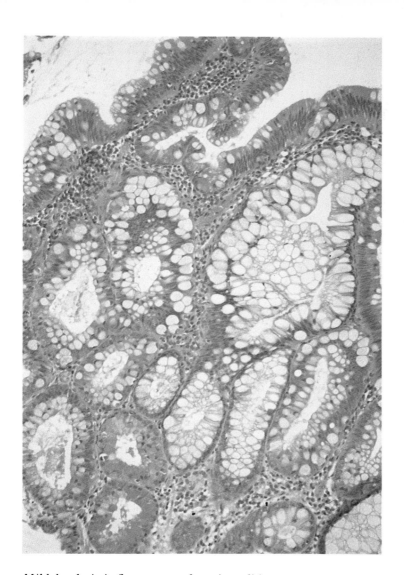

Mild dysplasia in flat mucosa, ulcerative colitis

The crypts show mild distortion with papillary infolding, branching and crowding. There is Paneth cell metaplasia.

H&E. ×160.

Fig. 124

Mild dysplasia in flat mucosa, ulcerative colitis

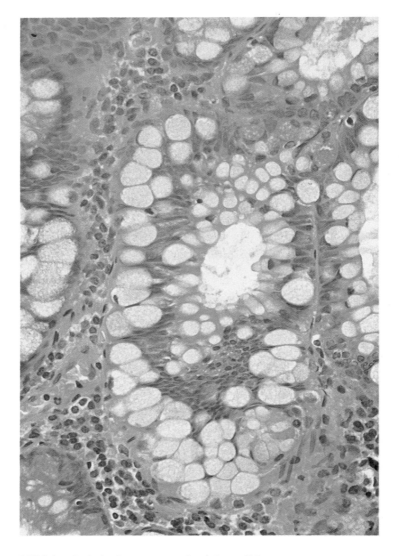

Mild dysplasia in flat mucosa, ulcerative colitis

Goblet cell inversion (dislocation, dystrophy) has resulted in a 'two cell layer' effect. The nuclei show only very slight enlargement and crowding.

H&E. ×400.

Fig. 125
*Moderate aysplasia in
flat mucosa, ulcerative
colitis*

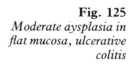

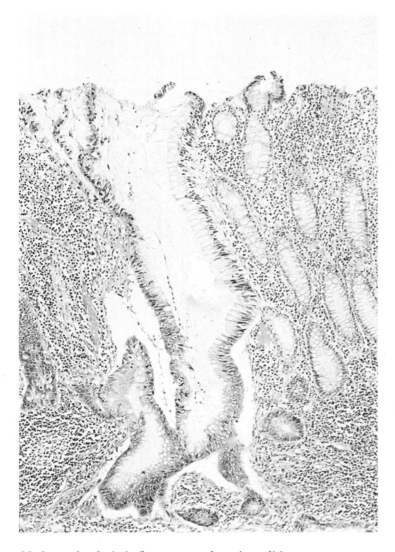

Moderate dysplasia in flat mucosa, ulcerative colitis

The crypt on the left is widened and lined by tall mucous cells. The crypt base region shows irregular branching (see Fig. 126).

H&E. ×100.

Fig. 126
Moderate dysplasia in flat mucosa, ulcerative colitis

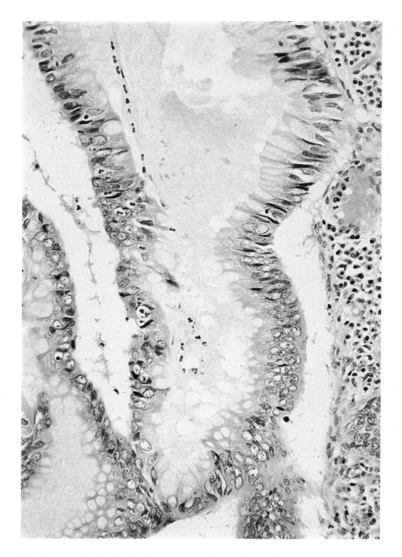

Moderate dysplasia in flat mucosa, ulcerative colitis

The nuclei of the crypt base region are enlarged, pleomorphic and pseudostratified. Mucus secretion is reduced. The lesion, which was associated with an underlying carcinoma, would be regarded as high grade dysplasia in the two-grade system.

H&E. ×250.

Fig. 127

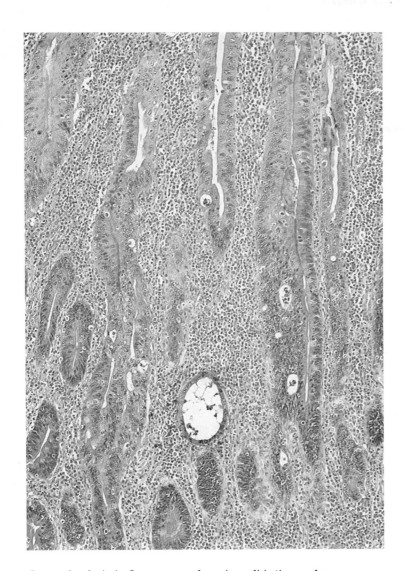

Severe dysplasia in flat mucosa, ulcerative colitis (incomplete maturation pattern)

The mucosa is greatly thickened and inflamed. The crypts are straight, but reveal architectural abnormalities including intra-epithelial cysts. They are lined by eosinophilic cells with hyperchromatic, basal nuclei. This variant of dysplasia shows features of incomplete maturation or basal cell hyperplasia (see Fig. 128). Carcinoma (not shown) usually arises from the crypt base region and is poorly differentiated.

H&E. ×100.

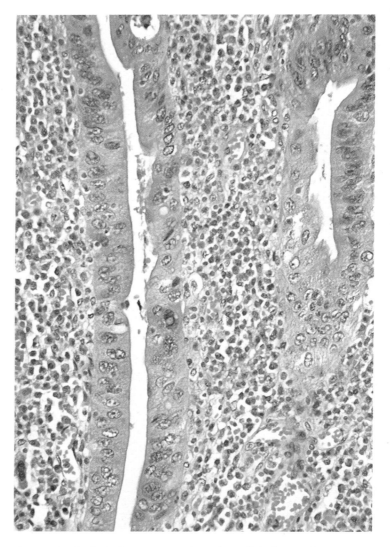

*Severe dysplasia in flat mucosa, ulcerative colitis (incomplete
maturation pattern)*

At higher magnification, the upper crypt epithelium shown in
Fig. 127 includes eosinophilic columnar cells but no normal
goblet cells. The nuclei are vesicular with a coarse nuclear
membrane and prominent nucleoli. They show focal loss of
polarity. The appearances are reminiscent of regenerative change
(see Fig. 116), but there is little active inflammation. In the
context of the low power field (Fig. 127), the changes are
interpreted as moderate to severe dysplasia (high grade in the
two-grade system).

H&E. ×250.

Fig. 129
*Moderate dysplasia in
flat mucosa, ulcerative
colitis (serrated pattern)*

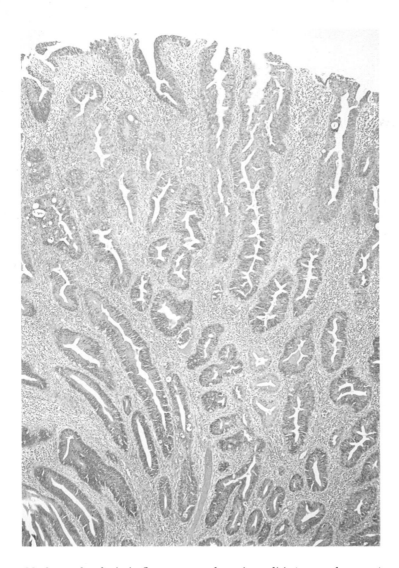

Moderate dysplasia in flat mucosa, ulcerative colitis (serrated pattern)

The mucosa is thickened and shows unbranched tubules with serrated contours—reminiscent of a hyperplastic polyp (see Fig. 130).

H&E. ×40.

Fig. 130

*Moderate dysplasia in
flat mucosa, ulcerative
colitis (serrated pattern)*

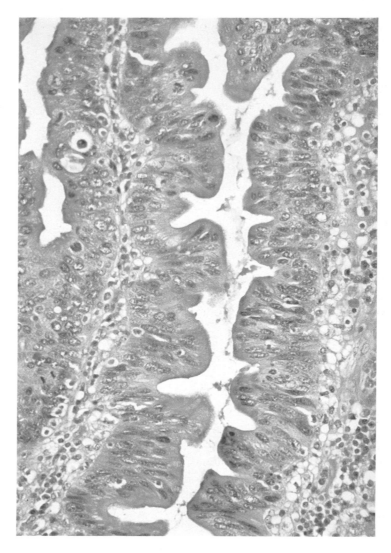

Moderate dysplasia in flat mucosa, ulcerative colitis (serrated pattern)

Nuclei are ovoid, hyperchromatic and pseudostratified, but
polarity is retained. In a two-grade system the changes would
probably be acceptable as an example of low grade dysplasia.

H&E. ×250.

Fig. 131
*Severe dysplasia in flat
mucosa, ulcerative
colitis*

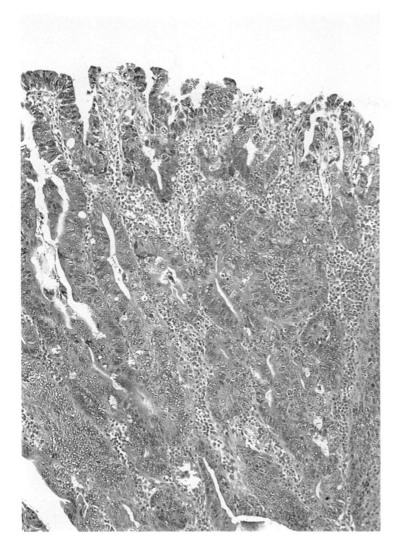

Severe dysplasia in flat mucosa, ulcerative colitis

The crypts show irregular branching and back-to-back
arrangements.

H&E. ×100.

Fig. 132
*Severe dysplasia in flat
mucosa, ulcerative
colitis*

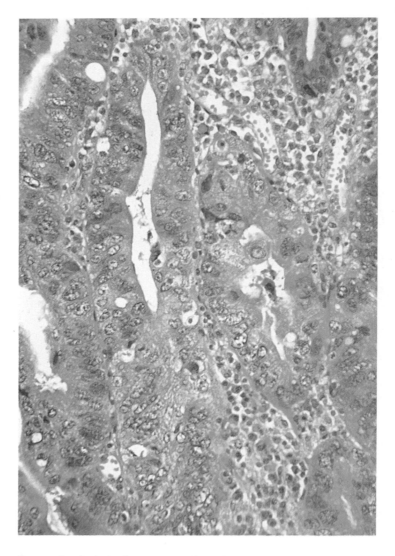

Severe dysplasia in flat mucosa, ulcerative colitis

The nuclei are hyperchromatic and show marked variation in size
and shape. Polarity is lost. An atypical mitotic figure is included.

H&E. ×250.

Fig. 133
*Dysplasia in
ureterosigmoidostomy*

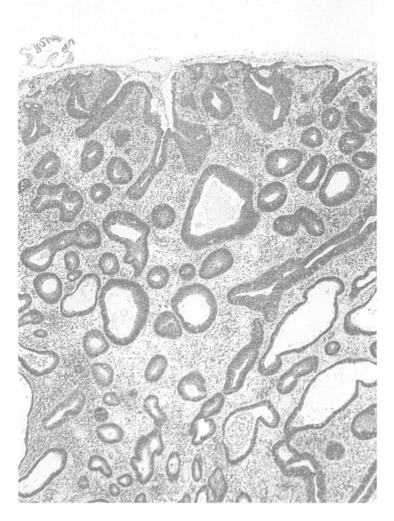

Dysplasia in ureterosigmoidostomy

The branching tubules set in an oedematous stroma invite
comparison with a regenerative or a juvenile polyp (Fig. 104). The
tubular epithelium shows the changes of mild to moderate
dysplasia.

H&E. ×40.

Fig. 134
Normal colorectal mucosa

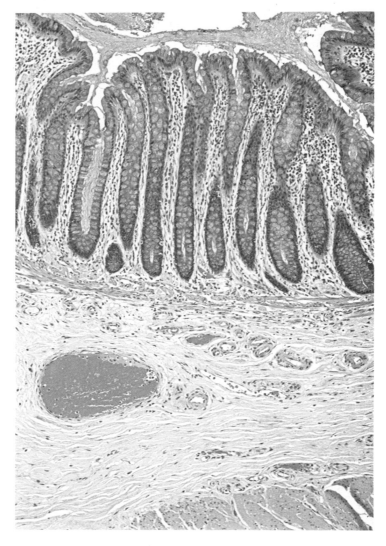

Normal colorectal mucosa

The crypts are simple, unbranched tubular structures.

H&E. ×100.

Fig. 135
*Normal colorectal
mucosa (mucins)*

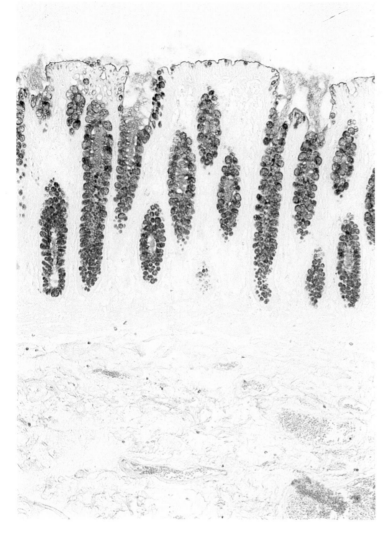

Normal colorectal mucosa (mucins)

The goblet cells secrete sulphomucins (brown) though small
amounts of sialomucin (blue) are present in the upper crypts and
surface epithelium.

High iron diamine/Alcian blue. ×100.

Fig. 136
Transitional mucosa,
colorectum

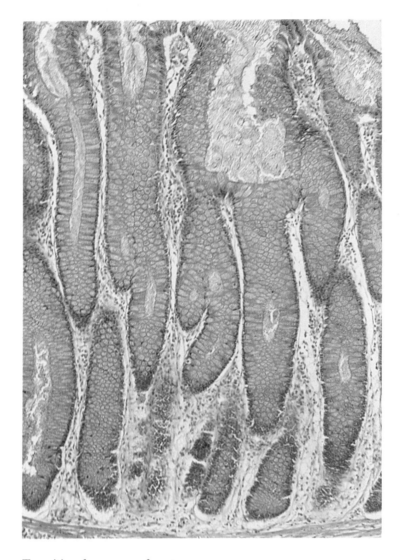

Transitional mucosa, colorectum

The mucosa is thickened and the crypts are branched and lined by tall mucous cells.

H&E. ×100.

Fig. 137
Transitional mucosa,
colorectum (mucins)

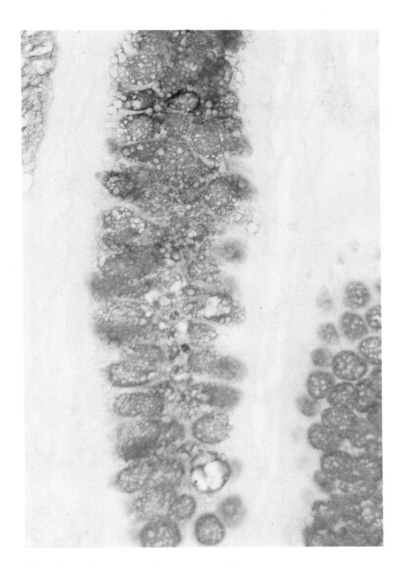

Transitional mucosa, colorectum (mucins)

Goblet cells secrete sialomucin (blue). Intervening immature mucous cells secrete small amounts of sulphomucin (brown).

High iron diamine/Alcian blue. ×100.

Fig. 138
Mild dysplasia, anal canal

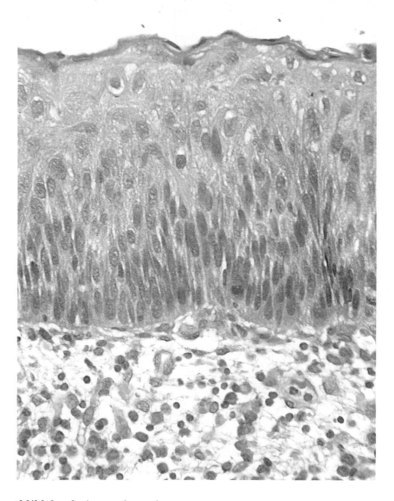

Mild dysplasia, anal canal

The epithelium is acanthotic, and atypical basal cells with enlarged hyperchromatic nuclei occupy the lower third. Above this level, maturation is little disturbed.

H&E. ×400.

Fig. 139
*Moderate dysplasia,
anal canal*

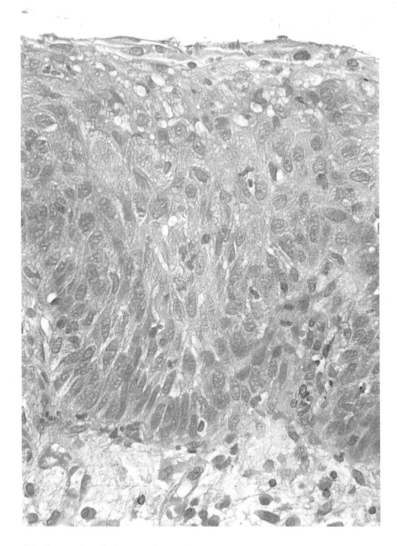

Moderate dysplasia, anal canal

The epithelium is thickened and atypical basal cells with enlarged, pleomorphic nuclei occupy the lower two thirds.

H&E. ×400.

Fig. 140
*Severe dysplasia, anal
canal*

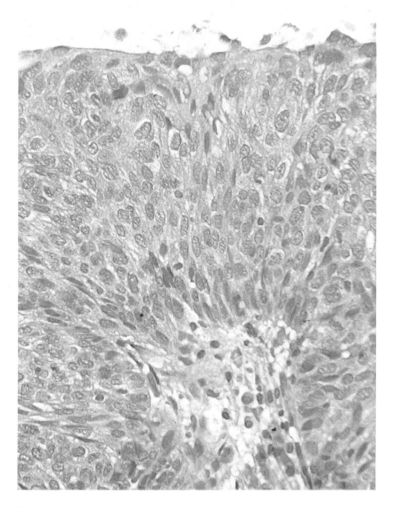

Severe dysplasia, anal canal

Atypical basal cells, with enlarged pleomorphic nuclei, occupy the
entire thickness of the acanthotic epithelium. There is only a hint
of cytoplasmic maturation.

H&E. ×400.

Fig. 141
Dysplasia, anal margin

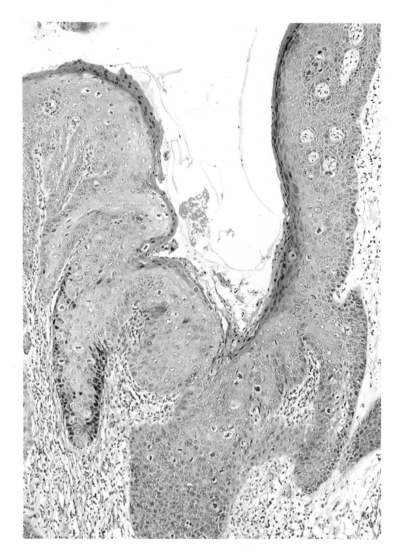

Dysplasia, anal margin

The epidermis is thickened with elongated rete ridges and there is a chronic inflammatory infiltrate in the superficial dermis (see Fig. 142).

H&E. ×100.

Fig. 142
Dysplasia, anal margin

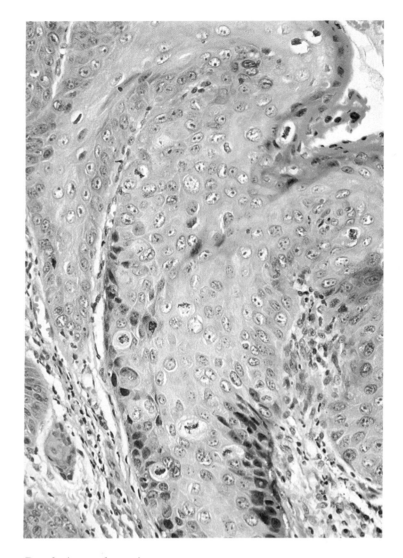

Dysplasia, anal margin

The nuclei are enlarged, vesicular and pleomorphic and there are numerous mitotic figures. Parakeratosis is present. Such severe nuclear atypia in the presence of cytoplasmic maturation is observed in Bowen's disease.

H&E. ×250.

Fig. 143
*Condyloma
acuminatum, anal
margin*

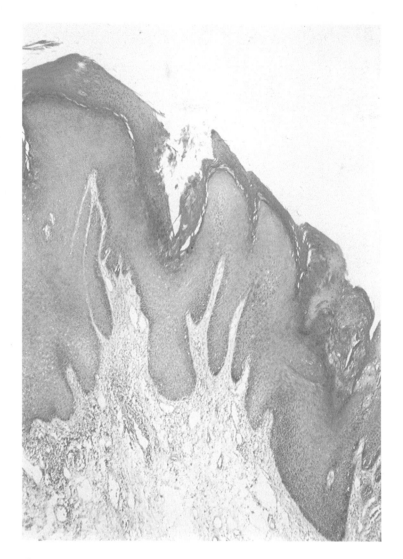

Condyloma acuminatum, anal margin

There is acanthosis, papillomatosis and parakeratosis. A characteristic acuminate or saw-tooth contour is formed.

H&E. ×40.

Fig. 144
*Condyloma
acuminatum, anal
margin*

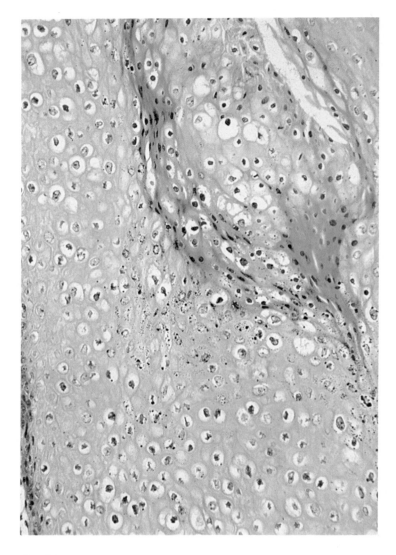

Condyloma acuminatum, anal margin

Characteristic vacuolation of the epidermal cells is shown.

H&E. ×250.

Fig. 145
*Giant condyloma, anal
margin*

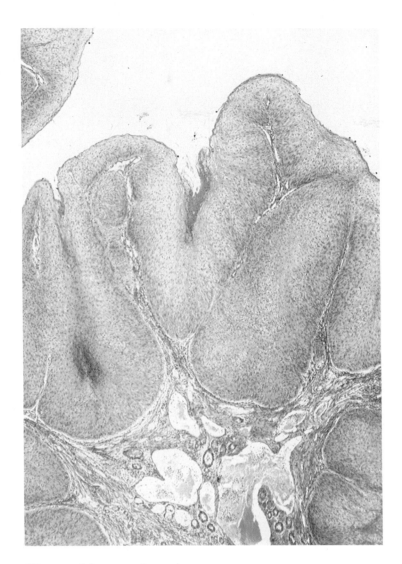

Giant condyloma, anal margin

There is acanthosis, papillomatosis and hyperkeratosis. The
tumour infiltrates with a broad front, characterized by the
formation of club-shaped epithelial processes. The underlying
dermis shows marked chronic inflammation (see Fig. 146).

H&E. ×60.

Fig. 146
Giant condyloma, anal margin

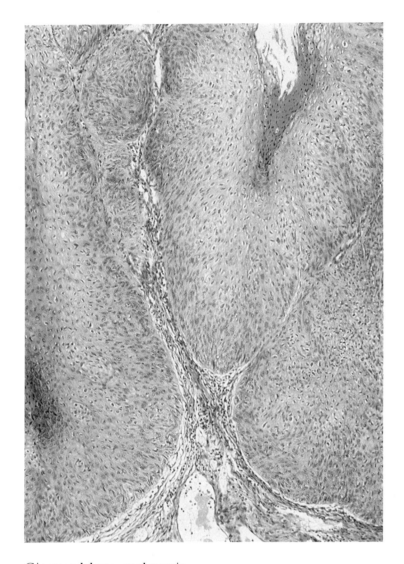

Giant condyloma, anal margin

The tumour is extremely well differentiated, belying its locally aggressive behaviour. Cell vacuolation is not present, but has been described within this family of tumours, suggesting a viral aetiology and a possible relationship with the more common condyloma acuminatum.

H&E. ×100.

Fig. 147
*Paget's disease, anal
margin*

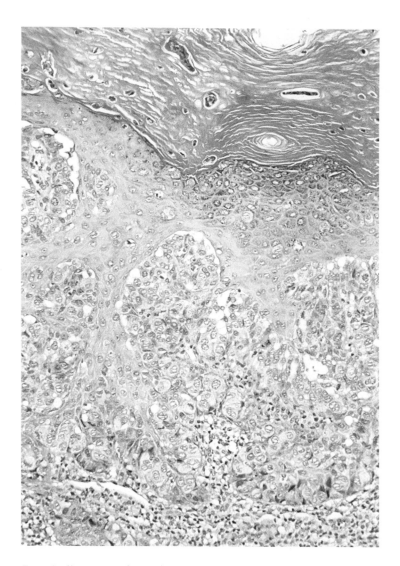

Paget's disease, anal margin

The epidermis is infiltrated with groups of large pale cells with
vesicular nuclei. These cells secrete sialomucin. There is overlying
hyperkeratosis and the lesion presented as a white plaque.

H&E. ×250.

Fig. 148
*Bowenoid papulosis,
anal margin*

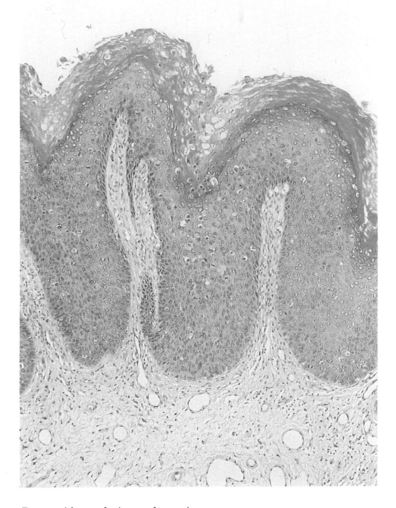

Bowenoid papulosis, anal margin

There is acanthosis, elongation of the rete ridges and hyperkeratosis (see Fig. 149).

H&E. ×100.

Fig. 149
*Bowenoid papulosis,
anal margin*

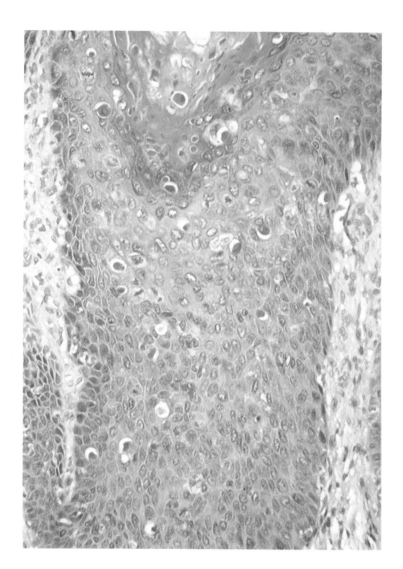

Bowenoid papulosis, anal margin

Scattered throughout the epidermis are small, dyskeratotic cells and large pale cells. The latter show mitotic activity. This results in a 'salt and pepper' appearance.

H&E. ×250.

Index of Precancerous Lesions and Conditions